# Critical approaches to ageing and later life

# Critical approaches to ageing and later life

Edited by
**ANNE JAMIESON**
**SARAH HARPER**
**CHRISTINA VICTOR**

Open University Press
Buckingham • Philadelphia

Open University Press
Celtic Court
22 Ballmoor
Buckingham
MK18 1XW

and
1900 Frost Road, Suite 101
Bristol, PA 19007, USA

First Published 1997

A catalogue record of this book is available from the British Library

ISBN 0 335 19725 6 (pbk)  0 335 19726 4 (hbk)

**Library of Congress Cataloging-in Publication Data**
Critical approaches to ageing and later life/edited by Anne
  Jamieson, Sarah Harper, Christine Victor.
        p.  cm.
    Chiefly based on papers presented at the 1994 Annual Conference of
the British Society of Gerontology.
    Includes bibliographical references and index.
    ISBN 0-335-19726-4 (hbk)      ISBN 0-335-19725-6 (pbk)
    1. Gerontology – Great Britain – Congress.   2. Aging – Social
aspects – Great Britain – Congresses.   3. Aged – Great Britain – Social
conditions – Congresses.   I. Jamieson. Anne.   II. Harper, Sarah.
III. Victor, Christina R.   IV. British Society of Gerontology.
Conference (1994)
HQ1064.G7C75   1997
305.26 – dc21                                                               97-568
                                                                              CIP

Typeset by Type Study, Scarborough
Printed in Great Britain by St Edmundsbury Press, Bury St Edmunds, Suffolk

To Glenda Laws

# Contents

**Part III: Concluding analysis**

# List of contributors

Andrew Achenbaum, Professor, Institute of Gerontology and Department of History, University of Michigan, Ann Arbor.

Andrew Blaikie, Senior Lecturer, Department of Sociology, University of Aberdeen.

Ken Blakemore, Lecturer in Social Policy, University of Wales, Swansea.

Bill Bytheway, Lecturer in Sociology, University of Wales, Swansea.

Eileen Fairhurst, Senior Lecturer, Department of Health Care Studies, Manchester Metropolitan University.

Sarah Harper, Member of the Wellcome Institute for the History of Medicine, University of Oxford.

Mike Hepworth, Reader, Department of Sociology, University of Aberdeen.

Paul Higgs, Lecturer, Unit of Medical Sociology, University College, London.

Anne Jamieson, Lecturer in Gerontology , Birkbeck College, University of London.

Margot Jefferys, Visiting Professor, King's College London.

Julia Johnson, Lecturer in Health and Social Welfare, Open University.

Joanna Latimer, Senior Research Fellow, Department of Nursing and Midwifery, Keele University.

Glenda Laws, (until her death in 1996) Associate Professor, Department of Geography, Pennsylvania State University.

David Troyansky, Associate Professor, Department of History, Texas Technical University.

Christina Victor, Senior Lecturer, St George's Hospital Medical School, University of London.

Hannah Zeilig, Research student, Age Concern Institute of Gerontology, King's College London.

ANNE JAMIESON, SARAH HARPER AND
CHRISTINA VICTOR

# Introduction

Our aim, in producing this book, has been to gather into one volume a wide range of contributions towards conceptual, if not theoretical, developments in social gerontology. Our hope is to challenge the notion that gerontology is a narrow discipline obsessed with enumerating the consequences for society of population ageing and with a research perspective which is dominated by the empiricist biomedical approach.

The book is divided into two parts. The chapters in Part I are primarily reflections on what *gerontology* is or should be, and the value of different disciplines and approaches. Bytheway addresses directly the question of what could be the theoretical basis for social gerontology. He does so by deconstructing the concept of age and analysing its different dimensions and the relation between them. Achenbaum reflects on the state of gerontology in the USA, and on what is entailed in what he calls critical gerontology. Blakemore offers a critical review of writing on cultural aspects of ageing, as represented by articles in *Ageing and Society*. He finds it wanting, in that the notion of ethnicity is generally used in relation to minority experiences. He proposes ways in which gerontology could develop insight by applying the concept of ethnicity to majorities. The following two chapters focus on the contributions of specific disciplines. Thus Zeilig discusses whether (fictional) literature can have more than merely illustrative value for the gerontologist. Troyansky writes from the historian's perspective and reviews a vast amount of historical research into ageing and cultural representations of old age. He comments on the changing and often conflicting 'findings' of historians, which cast doubt on the idea that history can 'correct' memory. He considers the merits of oral history and how history and gerontology have a common interest in the memory of older people. The position of memory in gerontological research is explored further by Fairhurst, who argues for a view of older people's memory as discourse to be studied in its own right, rather than as subjective representations to be judged against some 'real' events. An area in which interest has been growing is fictional literature and the ways in which this can contribute to an understanding of ageing issues.

The chapters in Part II represent a variety of ways in which concepts and theory can be applied in gerontology. Like the chapters in Part I, they suggest ways forward for gerontology, but more indirectly, through examples of *analyses of aspects of age and later life*. Jefferys addresses issues of inter-generational relations in the family and in work relations. She does so by putting her own personal account into a broader context of sociological theory. Laws presents an analysis of the meaning of retirement as it is manifested in the discourse around the Sun City retirement communities in the USA. She writes from a geographer's perspective and argues how a focus on space and spatial relations can provide insight into social relations. Blaikie and Hepworth focus on visual images related to ideas of old age and the status of older people. In their analysis of Victorian paintings and photographs they discuss ways in which such images should and should not be interpreted. Higgs discusses recent developments in social policy in Britain, and against this background, calls for a reassessment of the theory of structured dependency. Johnson and Bytheway discuss relations between the professional carers and the older people in institutional settings, as they are depicted in photographs. Their discussion is based on the view that photographs can both be reflective of and influence care practices. Care practices are also the focus of Latimer, who analyses the discourse of professionals in an acute hospital setting. Issues of bodily decline and death are discussed by Harper, who presents a feminist, critical assessment of concepts in this area.

In the final part of the book – Part III – we consider the contributions as a whole, in an attempt to draw out some of the current issues in gerontology. We focus on two different debates. The first debate relates to *epistemological issues*. This includes questions of the strengths and limitations of different *disciplinary perspectives* in gerontology, but perhaps even more importantly, it raises issues which cut across the disciplinary boundaries. Thus this volume highlights two specific debates, one around the nature of *critical gerontology*, and the other around *postmodernism*. As editors we have deliberately taken a pluralist position and assembled contributions which together represent a number of different, often conflicting, epistemological viewpoints.

The second set of debates we highlight centre on substantive *issues of ageing and later life*. The chapters in this book touch upon a wide range of questions, and we focus first on concepts related to ageing and later life in general, such as the meaning of *retirement* and the impact of consumerism on the notion of *structured dependency*. We also consider some aspects of *inter-generational relations* and the *politics* of ageing. Second, we address some of the issues and concepts associated with frailty and the end of life: the role of *health and social services*, concepts of the *declining body* and attitudes to *death*.

We believe that this book is testimony to the growing interest in theoretical issues in gerontology in Britain and elsewhere. The idea for the book arose from the 1994 Annual Conference of the British Society of Gerontology (BSG). Many papers were offered, and the sessions on this theme were very well attended. As conference organizers we decided with the BSG that a book on conceptual issues would be timely. In addition to chapters developed from papers presented at this conference, a number of other contributions were invited, to cover some of this diverse field, including perspectives from North America. The interest in ageing has offered opportunities for scholars to move outside and across traditional disciplinary boundaries, and this collection illustrates very well the multidisciplinary and interdisciplinary nature of gerontology.

We would like to thank all authors for what we trust will be welcomed as a set of stimulating contributions towards further developments in gerontological discourse.

# PART 1

# Reflections on gerontology

BILL BYTHEWAY

# Talking about age: the theoretical basis of social gerontology

There is a concern that, in the development of social gerontology, theory has been neglected. Much of the theory that is discussed derives from other disciplines and often makes dubious assumptions about the nature of age itself. In this chapter I have endeavoured to clarify some of the basic concepts that might concern a gerontological theorist.

In the demarcation of the territorial rights of academic disciplines, childhood and early life have been cornered largely by developmental psychologists and educationists, so that *in practice* we have to accept that gerontology is primarily about adulthood and later life. I would argue, however, that *in theory* we have to begin with an interest in age that is unconstrained by any division of the life course. To do otherwise would be to start from a position that ensured that gerontological theory reinforced certain fundamental prejudices. For example, although much has been gained from research that has focused on the changing position of 'elderly people' in society and on how 'old age' itself has become a social construction in the development of welfare policies, the repeated focus of gerontological research upon 'elderly people' and 'old age' has imbued these words with a kind of ontological truth (Bytheway 1995: 125).

Gubrium and Wallace (1990) have argued that theories of age have to build upon language, and upon the study of how people – including gerontologists – talk about age. They begin with the question 'who theorizes age?':

> not just professional social gerontologists theorise age; we all do to the extent that we set about the task of attempting to understand the whys and wherefores of growing old. It is argued that when the proprietary bounds of gerontological theorising are set aside striking parallels can be found between the everyday theorising of ordinary men and

women concerned with ageing and their more celebrated gerontological peers.

(Gubrium and Wallace 1990: 132)

Given this approach, it is possible to address the question: how do we refer or
allude to age in our everyday lives? It is in how we make reference to age, in
describing what we know and how we feel about it, that we conceptualize it.
One unavoidable consequence of this approach is that theories are ethno-
centric. This chapter, couched in the English language, draws upon my experience of how ideas about age are discussed in the UK in the latter part of the
twentieth century, both in gerontology and in everyday theorizing.

I have developed my argument by drawing upon two kinds of discourse.
The first concerns the articulation of ideas about how age is measured (Bytheway 1990) and experienced (Bytheway 1996). In preparing the first unit of the
Open University course 'An Ageing Society' (Gearing and Bytheway 1994), I
identified and distinguished six different ways in which students might
respond to this challenge. I summarized each as a basic question that – theoretically – could be asked of an individual:

• *Chronology*. How old are you chronologically?
• *Description*. What words would you use to describe how old you are?
• *Relations*. How is your experience of ageing being affected by other people?
• *Body*. How are observable changes in your body affecting your sense of ageing?
• *Pressures*. How is your experience of ageing being affected by social expec-
  tations and institutional regulations regarding age?
• *Biography*. How do you view your past and your future?

The second kind of discourse that I have considered is the casual description of an absent third party: ways in which people might describe or allude
to the age of an acquaintance. In the following argument I use the example
of Henry, a fictional acquaintance who has just decided to emigrate to South
Africa. I explore different ways in which his age and that of others might be
raised in ordinary conversation, and how this information might be related
to his decision to emigrate. I make the assumption that in Britain in the 1990s,
it would be odd if, in an extended but ordinary conversation about Henry's
decision, there were to be no reference or allusion to his age.

If Henry was introduced in person, his appearance would be sufficient to
indicate his approximate age. But in his absence, an introductory reference to
him – in conversation or in writing – would often include some more explicit
reference to his age in order that the introduction appears complete. In the
following, I explore different ways in which his age might feature in conversations among his acquaintances, and set this in the context of the six questions listed above.

## Chronology

Have you heard? Henry's decided to emigrate to South Africa. Quite a
decision for someone in his early sixties!

In late twentieth-century Britain, from the time we learn to count and to appreciate the annual cycle, we recognize that age and birthdays are things that children have in common with adults. Thus, in our early socialization prior to entry into schools, we acquire a powerful understanding of the social significance of *chronological age*. This understanding persists as a lifelong interest (Bytheway 1995: 73–7).

Chronological age quantifies the time between birth and the answering of the question. Thus chronological age is essentially a matter of measuring the distance between two points in historical time (Alheit 1994). Gerontologists occasionally describe chronological age as being less significant than other aspects of age. More commonly, however, there is some recognition that there is no satisfactory alternative as an indicator of the ageing process (Shock 1987). Implicit in this recognition is the idea that because chronological age itself cannot *cause* change, it is the ageing process, not chronological age, that gerontologists seek to study. Arguably, the same conceptualization applies in ordinary discourse. For example, it is difficult to imagine anyone seriously believing that Henry has made his decision to emigrate simply and solely because of the number of years that have passed since he was born.

Nevertheless, in understanding the significance of Henry's decision, chronological age would be considered important for four reasons. First, chronological age is the basis of many powerful expectations: 'A man in his early sixties should be thinking about easing up, not starting a new life in a distant country.' Second, it produces a form of equivalence: 'He's less than a year older than my father and he's never moved for forty years.' Third, it orders people according to historical experience: 'Henry was only seven when he was last in South Africa. It was still part of the Empire then, wasn't it?' Fourth, it is the basis of all kinds of institutional categorization: 'Cheap flights to Jo'burg. Exclusive to the over 50s.' It is for these four reasons that chronological age should feature in a theoretical account of age.

## Description

> Henry, old? Well, I know he took his early retirement last year but even so I wouldn't call him old.

All sorts of words are used in describing age, but there are four broad categories that predominate.

- Words which relate explicitly to age: middle-aged; teenager; old.
- Words which are less direct and involve social values and statuses but which, nevertheless, relate primarily to ideas about age: mature; grown-up; baby.
- Other social statuses that indirectly imply age: schoolchild; married; working; student; retired; pensioner.
- Colloquial phrases, many of which are clearly ageist: past it; grey; in the prime of life; just a big kid; going ga-ga; still young at heart.

All of these words and phrases are alternatives to chronological age in describing the age of a person. They are often used to specify rather more precisely the age status of an individual, often as an elaboration upon chronological age: 'Really, at heart, Henry's still just a big kid.' Most of these descriptive words are adjectival, implicitly casting the individual into a category:

> 'So you wouldn't call Henry old?'
> 'No.'
> 'So what is "old"?'
> 'Well . . .'
> 'What about his mother?'
> 'Oh, definitely. She's 92, she's very old.'
> 'And what about his older sister, Daphne?'
> 'Well, she's getting on too. She's over 70, I think, and so, yes, I suppose I'd call her old too.'

Although this exchange includes all kinds of subtle connotations, the fact is that through the use of words both Henry's mother and sister are being included in the category 'old', whereas Henry is not. In this limited sense, the outcome of this exchange is that they are being perceived to be equivalent to each other in age and he is being perceived to be different.

Through scientific study and bureaucratic refinements, any word can come to be given a precise technical definition and applied on the basis of agreed criteria. Institutionalized categorization that is based on such keywords can have real consequences for the lives of persons so assessed. For example, a report to the local authority housing committee might have begun: 'In the context of this report, people over the age of 75 are referred to as "elderly".' As a direct result of this, Henry's mother and a number of other people over 75 years of age became residents of what is specifically called 'a home for the elderly'. Indeed, Henry may walk past a sign saying 'Eventide Home for the Elderly' as he visits his mother to tell her of his decision. In this way, through constant usage, simple adjectives such as 'elderly' come to acquire a wide range of subtle meanings and associations in the public arena, in the technical discourse of scientists and bureaucrats and, eventually, in ordinary conversation.

## Relations

> Well another reason I wouldn't call Henry old is that his youngest daughter, Polly, is still only 17.

It is often the case that although we do not know the precise age of acquaintances, we do know the ages of their children. People sometimes avoid revealing their own age by referring to the ages of their children. It is, moreover, a way of associating oneself with youthfulness. The famous advertisement selling facecream, for example, uses this ploy: 'How old am I? Well, my daughter is 17 and she uses [this cream] too!'

Children are age-graded. The educational system is based on an annual incremental approach to child development. As children move up each year from one class to another, progressing numerically upwards from the first to the sixth form, they are assessed against age-specific standards. This ensures that parents become age conscious – aware of the passing of the years as their children graduate one year at a time through school. At no other time in life are we graded so precisely or so publicly according to our age. The growth of children on all sorts of biological, psychological and educational dimensions is closely related to chronological age, so it would be surprising if this were ignored. But taking account of age in monitoring the development of children is different from providing education to age-graded and numbered classes.

The consequence of this way of organizing the provision of early education is that the parents (and grandparents) of children who happen to be in a particular class share many age-related experiences as their children move through the school. Moreover, as a result of there being a national education system, they also share with parents of children in other schools many of the experiences that are characteristic of parenting a child of the same age.

Henry, for example, may be compared with other fathers of daughters of 17 and many pertinent similarities and differences might be noted. These are relevant not just because of what it is for Polly to be 17 years of age (and for her to have a father in his early sixties), but also because of what it is for Henry to be the parent of a 17-year-old. For example, it may be that his lifestyle and everyday routines seem more oriented to his daughter's age than to his own. Similarly, it may be that his decision to emigrate to South Africa is thought to be connected to the prospect of Polly, his youngest child, becoming an independent adult – perhaps as old as he was when he first travelled round the globe.

Age relations may be used not just to amplify the age of the individual; they are the basis of an alternative mapping of age, one that is not so closely linked to personal biography. 'He must have been over 40 when Polly was born! My Dad was only 21 and he still hasn't reached 40!' In this way, differences in chronological age are often conflated with the concept of generation. Two different aspects of generation need to be distinguished. One relates to family structure and the fact that at birth everyone has two parents, both of an 'adult' age. In the social identification of parents (allowing for all the complications of mortality, adoptions, fostering, hospital errors, in vitro fertilization and so on), we all acquire a certain knowledge of, or beliefs about, the identities – and in particular the ages – of our two parents. The various lives of grandparents, parents, children and grandchildren, building upon relationships established at birth and upon the power of the family as a social institution, serve to place people in a generational context which determines much of their experience and expectations of ageing.

Polly's friends can compare Henry with their parents. Probably (certainly in the UK in the 1990s), he will be conspicuously older than most of their fathers, and some may note that he is old enough to be her grandfather. These kinds of perceptions may have all sorts of consequences for the experience that he and Polly have of age.

Similar relational indicators of age affect other networks of generational relationships, such as those between teachers and students. In all these social relations, the pattern of regeneration and the organization of inheritance and succession should be central to a theory explaining the significance of age relations. 'The thing about Henry is that he is part of the post-war never-had-it-so-good generation. Daphne, in contrast, is a child of the depression. She had to raise her two children on her own during the war.' The other aspect of generation that needs to be distinguished is the cultural. Henry and Daphne may be perceived to be of different generations, for example, if they subscribe to the cultural values that are associated with different historical cohorts. Of course, this begs the questions: with what different experiences do different cohorts associate, and what is meant by associate? No one would ask Henry and Daphne to register themselves as members of one generation or another. The categorization remains implied rather than implemented.

In both respects – family and culture – our association with the idea of a generation produces a sense of ageing, either through shared activities and memories, or as members of our generation pass through various age-associated life events: marriage, parenthood, retirement, death.

## Body

> Henry has looked after himself. What little hair he's got may be white, but he's kept himself in trim.

In our first years, as we grow rapidly in height and weight, we learn that the body changes in appearance as we age. Even though changes are not so predictable in later life, there is a range of signs to which we are all sensitive: the colour and loss of hair, the texture of the skin, the shape of the body, agility, sight and so on. Increasingly these physical changes are seen to constitute the essence of age, and by resisting or denying at least some of these changes, we may imagine that we can 'put off' age (Turner 1995). But we know that, in reality, the sight of our body betrays all but the details.

Henry, feeling that he is visibly older than all the fathers of Polly's friends, may have been tempted to present a more youthful image by concealing the state of his hair with a toupee. To those who knew him (not least to Polly), his reasons would be all too apparent and so all sorts of comments would have been made about his apparent sensitivity over age. So he may have decided to keep fit and active instead, and not worry too much about his hair.

Bodily indicators of age in adulthood are comparable with the symptoms of illness. Stiff limbs, for example, can be interpreted as a sign of either ill-health or age. Many diseases are diagnosed through the recognition of such signs. In the same way, age is recognized in part by physical signs. No matter whether we interpret changes in the body in terms of age or ill-health, we are inclined, in accordance with dominant cultural values, to judge these changes systematically and negatively. We are acutely aware that a wide range of changes indicate a decline in health. When they appear we expect the doctor to do something. We want to recover our health and to resume life as it was. We tend to think of age quite differently. Although we may resist it in the short term, we are taught that it is inevitable over the course of a lifetime. We are encouraged to 'age well' but never to 'fall ill well'.

Many of the signs of age, however, are similar to those of ill-health, and we often look to the doctor for treatment or advice. The health services encourage us to keep our bodies healthy and fit, and so those aspects of age that are judged negatively have been medicalized (Estes and Binney 1991). We are taught that, by 'looking after ourselves' and by following the guidance of health education, we can sustain an age-free image of health and well-being for much of our lives. But we are also led to expect a time to come when, due to age, this is no longer possible. As a result, we tend to view age negatively in much the same way as we view chronic illness.

## Pressures

> Henry is in his early sixties; he's had a full life. He's retired now and drawing his occupational pension. Polly hopes to go to university and so is still dependent on him. His mother's 92 and not as fit as she used to be. Don't you think Henry ought to stay in Britain where his family is?

Access to education, employment and care is largely restricted to certain age groups, both through institutional regulation and through social expectation. The law imposes age restrictions on many other aspects of life: sexual activity, marital status, legal liability, political activity, migration and so on.

A theory of age should account for the construction and institutional regulation of age categories. Henry's retirement and pension, his mother's need for care and Polly's access to a university education, are all heavily constrained by rules regarding age. Much of this draws upon and contributes to the dissemination of age stereotypes. For example, because most pensions are tied rigidly to age categories, the word 'pensioner' has come to refer not just to the receipt of a pension but to a more general age category, often as a synonym for 'old person'. In modern society, all forms of media play a part in the production of these models of age; advertisements and soap operas being only the most obvious.

Similarly, family life imposes expectations regarding the pattern of daily living of people of different ages, expectations that are often close to institutionalized regulation. A powerful vocabulary results, one that virtually dictates the patterning of everyday life over the 'normal' life course: infant, schoolchild, teenager, newly weds, young homeless, working life, mid-life crisis, empty nest, retirement, third-ager, pensioner, widow, terminal illness. The narrow definition of many of these age expectations enables us to comment on those who are early or late, younger or older; for example, about Henry being an 'older parent' and 'early retired'. In much of this, the emphasis that is placed upon maintaining continuity is often seen in terms of 'settling down': Henry, for example, has reached a point where some think he should settle down rather than start 'a new life' in South Africa.

## Biography

> Henry used to be a bank manager. Since he retired he's spent most of his time on the golf course. But now that he's put his house on the market, he's looking forward to his move to South Africa.

Age orientates us to our life course and, conversely, our biography reflects our age (Kohli 1986). To say that Henry 'used to be' a bank manager and that he now spends 'most of his time' on the golf course indicates fairly definitely that he is now 'retired'. In this association with time and time-consuming activities such as golf, the word 'retired' acquires a meaning that is divorced from the world of work. This simple biographical statement, using tense and referring to time, provides a vivid and concise image of current changes in Henry's life course, and from this it is not difficult to gain a sense of his age.

Earlier in his life Henry may have been seen to be a possible golf champion. Later on, settled in the bank, his successes and failures in furthering his career in banking will have been noted. Over time a growing biography developed, which accounted for what he had done and in what order, and for his changing future prospects. The dates of various past events come to be seen as critical turning points in this evolving biography, helping to explain how certain developments came to be. Later on, as retirement approached, his future may have seemed less important, and Henry's life may have been viewed rather more retrospectively, as if all the most significant events had happened, and as if what remained was for Henry to settle down, to indulge in his golf and to play his part in the continuing life of his family. Whatever the case, over the course of his life, the balance between what Henry can look back upon and what he can look forward to has steadily and inevitably changed, and this unfolding biography affects how his age is described and perceived.

In this view of age, the two critical orienting events in the life course are birth and death. It follows that one's birth is the event to which one's view of the past is referenced and, in a similar way, it is in the context of the changing prospects of death that one thinks of the future. In a literal sense, birth is our individual origin on the time dimension. We may have a clear sense of a continuing cultural history that flows past our own birthdate disregardingly, and likewise of a family history in which we make connections between our lives and those of our parents and grandparents and so on. But our personal experience of history is confined to personal recollection. From our childhood onwards we have experienced, discussed and contributed to the unfolding history of the worlds in which we have participated (Bytheway 1996). With age we accumulate this fund of personal experience and much of it can be enumerated in the same way as are birthdays: so many children, so many jobs, so many wars, so many books published, so many periods out of work, so many cars, so many marriages and so on. This cataloguing and enumeration of our past – typified for many of us perhaps by the formulation of our curricula vitae – is the way in which the past contributes to our sense of age. It is one way in which we can allude to our age.

Regarding the future, we can only bank on death and the intervening period: our time left. But, with regard to these two basic elements of the future, we can formulate expectations which, having a real impact upon our own view of our prospects, can lead to the most complex or the simplest of life plans.

'Henry. Why are you emigrating?'
'Well, I realized that, having retired, I was able to choose either to stay here, with my golf, my family and these familiar surroundings, or I could

start out afresh in South Africa. I weighed it all up, talked about it with Mother, Daphne and Polly, and decided: right I'm off.'

## Summary

Social gerontology needs a theoretical base which frees it from many of the restrictive and often ageist assumptions of contemporary culture, one which facilitates two simple objectives:

1 To gain a better understanding of how people experience and manage age over the course of their diverse lives.
2 To demonstrate how age is used in the formulation of expectations, in the regulation of rights and in the allocation of resources.

This base must include a clear conceptualization of age itself. In particular, its relationship to health, generation and social status needs to be more clearly understood. Like them, age is not quite as simple a concept as it first appears. My aim in this chapter has been to try to disentangle six different aspects: chronology, description, relations, body, pressures and biography. Apart from developing theory, this disaggregation may be useful for developing strategies in specific areas of gerontological research. For example, a study of ageing might relate to chronology, body and biography; a study of variations between different age groups to descriptions, relations and body; a study of how society conceptualizes age and regulates age groups to chronology, descriptions and pressures; a study of how age affects interpersonal relations to relations, pressures and biography.

## References

Alheit, P. (1994) Everyday time and life time, *Time and Society*, 3(3), 305.
Bytheway, B. (1990) Age, in S. Peace (ed.) *Researching Social Gerontology*. London: Sage.
Bytheway, B. (1995) *Ageism*. Buckingham: Open University Press.
Bytheway, B. (1996) The experience of later life, *Ageing and Society*, 16(5), 613–21.
Estes, C.L. and Binney, E.A. (1991) The biomedicalization of aging: dangers and dilemmas, in M. Minkler and C.L. Estes (eds) *Critical Perspectives on Aging*. Amityville, NY: Baywood, 117–34.
Gearing, B. and Bytheway, B. (1994) Ageism and Old Age, Unit 2, *An Ageing Society (K256)*. Milton Keynes: The Open University.
Gubrium, J. and Wallace, B. (1990) Who theorises age?, *Ageing and Society*, 10(2), 131–50.
Kohli, M. (1986) The world we forgot: a historical review of the life course, in V.W. Marshall (ed.) *Later Life: the Social Psychology of Aging*. London: Sage, 271–303.
Shock, N. (1987) Physiological age, in G.L. Maddox (ed.) *The Encyclopedia of Aging*. New York: Springer, 522–3.
Turner, B.S. (1995) Aging and identity: some reflections on the somatization of the self, in M. Featherstone and A. Wernick (eds) *Images of Aging: Cultural Representations of Later Life*. London: Routledge, 245–60.

# 2 W. ANDREW ACHENBAUM

# Critical gerontology

Like many others, researchers on ageing suffer from 'physics envy' (Keller 1982). Compared to physics (and chemistry, biology, economics, political science, psychology and sociology), the scientific study of ageing is a relatively 'young' field. Not only is gerontology immature in terms of longevity, but it lacks a firm theoretical foundation and unique methodologies. Researchers on ageing throughout the century have none the less confidently assured themselves that progress would be made if they emulated the 'hard' sciences, notably physics. As a result, gerontology's gatekeepers have been unabashedly scientistic as they tried to legitimize their area of expertise.

Establishing scientific criteria is difficult, however, in a field shaped by so many research perspectives. Gerontologists have different intellectual backgrounds: most were trained in highly specialized biomedical, behavioural and social scientific disciplines. Even among clinicians, foci vary; more nurses than physicians belong to the Gerontological Society of America. Negotiating common ground in a multidisciplinary endeavour is more problematic than in a department because experts employ divergent conventions and strategies to produce and disseminate knowledge. Some gerontologists advocate a live-and-let-live spirit in order to reduce rivalries and nurture a sense of community. Yet this tack dismays 'bench' scientists, who know that diffuseness is inimical to laboratory reductionism.

Recognizing the value of crossing disciplinary lines, gerontologists have been inclined for most of this century to endorse physicists' esteem for positivist logic and quantifiable measurements. They test and reject hypotheses. Their journals disseminate peer-reviewed papers that reduce complex phenomena to graphic charts. More like physicists than historians, researchers on ageing rely on straightforward language rather than nuanced evasions to convey ideas. At scientific gatherings, scholars probably invoke Sigmund Freud more than any other twentieth-century figure, but Albert Einstein represents the scientific ideal, and his successors have not hesitated to capitalize on the glory of his genius.

Gerontological 'physics envy' also affects how ageing-related projects are structured. Investigators realize that pay-offs are in 'big science' (Ziman 1994). Ever since the federal government underwrote teams of scientists to develop an atomic bomb in the Second World War, physicists have procured billions of dollars for large-scale teams of investigators to tackle highly sophisticated problems that promise to have profoundly significant applications. This led to the creation of all sorts of peer-review competition in the National Institutes of Health, National Science Foundation and other federal agencies, as well as in the private sector.

Paradoxically, gerontologists nowadays may actually be more wedded to positivism than physicists, who lately have been criticizing the ways that scientism thwarts creativity. Einstein himself worried about over-specialization in areas of quantum mechanics that relied unduly on theories that were obsolescent. 'Chaos theory' originated in the minds of physicists accustomed to thinking of complex systems of fluid dynamics (Glieck 1987). Does this mean that only 'mature' fields like physics can afford to scrutinize their own intellectual foundations at the risk of undermining them? No: domains (such as urban studies and computer science) emerging after the Second World War have also proven elastic enough to foster assaults on logical positivism, such as articulated by Thomas Kuhn and Imre Lakatos, among other philosophers of science. 'Critical theory' itself, after all, dates back at least to the 1930s: scholars associated with the so-called Frankfurt School began to bewail the wake of Hegelianism on human understanding. Max Horkheimer and his colleagues deplored the abstract separation of empirical research from philosophy, which did not allow for the significance of historically contingent developments. Within two decades, the Frankfurt School was deeply divided about the relevance and future of its original project and had begun to create autonomous clusters within the ranks (Honneth 1987).

The Frankfurt School's singular contribution was to affect the manner in which scholars analysed patterns of communication. Karl Mannheim and Jurgen Habermas set the stage for a self-reflexive stance in interpreting domain-specific ideas in a broad historical context. Adapting Marxist theories and notions borrowed from fields as disparate as the behavioural sciences and hermeneutics, scholars investigated 'turns' in intellectual discourse; they explored assumptions embedded in writers' arguments. Such self-reflexivity about the meanings of meaning and the language of discourse has, in no preordained or predictable fashion, often fed upon itself while inviting input from multiple, outside sources which transformed paradigms.

'Critical gerontology' shapes some investigations of ageing-related problems, but its influence thus far has been marginal. To substantiate this characterization, this chapter will unfold in ways that differ from 'standard' gerontological articles. The next section will trace three phases in feminist theory, which have profoundly transformed the ways that scholars in the humanities, social and behavioural fields, and even in some natural sciences, think about their evidence and interpret their data. I then survey the literature of ageing to determine the status of 'critical theory'. Finally, I propose that critical gerontology would be enhanced by incorporating more feminist theory, a theme reiterated by Harper later in this volume.

## The latest waves of feminism in academic discourse

Women's voices have long been expressed in scholarly treatises and intellectual exchanges. US women were challenging conventional wisdom (typically expressed by middle-class white males) before the founding of the Republic. Ann Hutchinson (1591–1643) sparked the antinomian controversy when she defied Puritan ministers with her views on divine revelation; Anne Bradstreet (1612–72) used poetry and elegies to convey new possibilities for comity in relations between the sexes during the colonial era. Abigail Adams urged her husband John 'to remember the ladies' as he and his fellow revolutionaries sought to frame a *novo ordo seclorum* (Salzman 1986). In the first decades of the nineteenth century, writers such as Hannah More and Lydia Maria Child transformed 'bonds of womanhood', premised on the perfectibility of women's moral being. The abolitionist movement at all levels was spearheaded by Northern and Southern women, many of whom gathered in Seneca Falls, New York in 1848 to rewrite the Declaration of Independence into a 'Declaration of Sentiments', to take account of women's right to marry, own property, work and enjoy other fruits of gender equality (Cott 1977; Cott and Pleck 1979).

Decades passed before provisions of the 1848 Seneca Falls Declaration became law, but there were advances in women's education beyond primary 'female departments' and seminaries. After 1870, a majority of high-school graduates were female. Vassar (1865), Wellesley and Smith (both 1875) and Bryn Mawr (1884) offered intellectual opportunities equal to those afforded to men at Harvard, Yale and Trinity; over a hundred coeducational colleges and universities had been founded by 1900 (Woloch 1991). Yet few women enjoyed equal status in the professions. More likely to teach grammar than conduct graduate seminars, women were encouraged to become nurses, not doctors; female physicians debated among themselves whether their gender gave them special healing powers, while denying them privileges in grand rounds or private practice (Rosenberg 1983; Morantz-Sanchez 1985).

The struggle for gender equality proceeded slowly during the first half of the twentieth century. While Amendment XIX (1920) declared that 'the right of citizens of the United States to vote shall be not be denied or abridged by the United States or by any State on account of sex', few women were elected to Congress or state houses before the New Deal. Nearly half of all college students in 1920 were women, but their percentages dropped for the next five decades. Research universities tended to exclude promising scholars who were not the right sex, race or religion. Gifted artists such as Edith Wharton and Georgia O'Keefe achieved international reputations, to be sure, and women of colour such as Zora Neale Hurston were integral to the Harlem Renaissance. But wealth, talent and patrons typically were not enough to enable women to gain access to the same opportunities that men assumed was their due.

Significant change came only with a revolutionary shift in consciousness during the post-war period. 'Gradually, without seeing it clearly for quite a while, I came to realize that something was very wrong with the way American women are trying to live their lives today,' wrote Betty Friedan in 1963. 'There was a strange discrepancy between the reality of our lives as women and the image to which we were trying to conform, the image that I came to call the feminine mystique. I wondered if other women faced this schizophrenic split, and what it meant' (Friedan 1963: 7). That same year, the Commission on the Status of Women issued a report documenting that women were denied equal rights. Congress took action. Lyndon Baines Johnson signed the 1964 Civil Rights Act, which guaranteed women as well as African-Americans greater opportunities. Enforcing gender equality became a public policy matter. Amidst the political ferment of the civil rights movement, a new wave of feminism affected all facets of American society.

Feminism swept higher education. The percentage of women attending professional schools soared, and curricula were modified to address gender issues. Disciplinary responses varied. Thanks to the influence of Margaret Mead and Ruth Benedict, and a long-standing focus on kinship networks, anthropologists early on attended to the cultural, social and biological significance of sex. An internal debate in psychology concerning women as objects and as subjects of analysis led to novel ways of 'exploring gender as noun and verb' (Fine and Gordon 1992: 1; Stacey and Thorne 1993). Sociology lagged, though by the early 1970s feminist perspectives were engendering new ways of thinking (Bernard 1973). Historians elaborated on the discrepancies between what they knew about women's history and what they discovered about gender inequalities in past times based on present-day circumstances. In virtually all disciplines arose radical feminists who demanded that theory and practice be woven along gender lines. Their manifesto made three interrelated points, which refocused the scholarly gaze: first, women have long been oppressed; second, women scholars must proclaim that 'the personal is the political'; and, third, they must engage in consciousness-raising activities that will transform their scholarship (Baym 1992; Stanley and Wise 1993).

Not surprisingly, scholars (mainly male) ridiculed the writings of radical feminists. The 'oppression' of women, they claimed, was exaggerated in models that rested on biological determinism or gender-laden cultural determinism. 'Feminist science is at best an antithesis to the distortion imposed by an excessively male-oriented perspective on human affairs' (Davidson 1988: 212). Critics deplored the anti-positivist bias in feminist writing. Assaults became more strident as conservative political ideologies displaced liberal rhetoric in the 1980s. George Gilder, Alan Bloom and Dinesh D'Souza attacked feminist arguments for undermining 'objective' analyses and substituting ephemeral works for classics.

Significantly, some of the nastiest criticisms of writers such as Simone de Beauvoir, Kate Millet, Germaine Greer and even Betty Friedan – stalwarts of the 1960s consciousness-raising movement – were levelled by feminists, who attacked the white, middle-class biases of the founding sisters. Feminist theory failed 'to recognize the embeddedness of its own assumptions within a specific historical context' (Nicholson 1990: 1–2). Responding to the charge, US feminist scholars made deliberate efforts to include the voices and experiences of lesbians, people of colour and others who hitherto had not been heard.

Scholars exercised greater care in presuming that 'gender' invariably should be privileged over 'class', 'race' or 'ethnicity' in the examination of inequalities and human relationships.

Feminist theory as well as empirical work by women underwent critical scrutiny which led to significant transformations in academic mores. US scholars established networks with peers in Europe and the Far East, subscribing to journals such as the marxist *Feminist Review* and *Women's Studies International Forum*, and publishing with British houses, such as Routledge, that were more receptive to radical scholarship than US firms. As intellectuals tried to incorporate the insights of such Continental theorists as Foucault, Bourdieu and Lacan in their writings, they also probed for gender biases: they did not want to repeat the mistake that the first wave of post-war feminists had made in not acknowledging the sexism embedded in Freud's scholarship (Kreiswirth and Cheetham 1990). Some critics went a step further, urging on epistemological grounds a remaking of the academy itself: *feminist sociology*, for instance, was to be 'not a sociology of gender, nor a sociology of women, but the remaking of the discipline in feminist terms' (Stanley and Wise 1993: 8).

As a result of this internal debate among women scholars, a second wave of feminism arose. 'Personal', direct experience remained key in feminist social science: 'If all our stories are indeed our own, if social research is largely autobiography, then the stories of this text are, of course, mine' (Fine 1992: xii; see also Stanley and Wise 1993). Yet the historical moment changed the political context. The Equal Rights Amendment was not ratified, but gender issues, ranging from abortion rights to labour-force discrimination to the plight of divorced mothers with children, remained at the political forefront. Amidst a conservative backlash, second-wave feminists supported a variety of practical reforms to promote justice. 'Feminist politics is not just a tolerable companion of feminist research but a necessary condition for generating less partial and perverse descriptions and explanations,' declared philosopher of science Sandra Harding in 1987. 'In a socially stratified society, the objectivity of the results of research is increased by political activism by and on behalf of oppressed, exploited and dominated groups' (Harding 1987). Sexual inequality, feminists realized, was one – not the only – problem besetting the nation.

Gains made in higher education mobilized the feminist cause. White women remained the most likely to have had twelve years of schooling between 1970 and 1991, but significantly the proportion of African-American women with high-school diplomas doubled during the period; women of Hispanic origin were not far behind. One-third of all women attending college were over the age of thirty, and the number of part-time students increased greater than the number of full-time students. A female member of the class of 1990 was twice as likely to be a biology major as her counterpart in the class of 1960; the number of business majors sextupled (Costello and Stone 1994).

Not only had women become an ever more diverse part of the (under)graduate population, but feminist thinking infused every discipline. New journals such as *Signs, Feminism & Psychology* and *Ms.* mixed politics and culture; mainstream quarterlies embraced radical perspectives. Feminism was far more interdisciplinary. Nearly everybody in the humanities and social sciences was talking about 'the postmodern turn'; feminists used the construct to challenge the vaunted 'objectivity' of unreflexive scientific research. 'A postmodernist reflection on feminist theory reveals disabling vestiges of essentialism while a feminist reflection on postmodernism reveals androcentrism and political naiveté,' observed Nancy Fraser and Linda Nicholson (1990: 20), critics who each held appointments in three departments. 'The ultimate stake of an encounter between feminism and postmodernism is the prospect of a perspective which integrates their respective strengths while eliminating their respective weaknesses.' Since the 1980s, feminists have crossed geographic boundaries too, borrowing ideas from below the equator as well as on the European continent.

## Insinuating a self-reflexive mode of discourse into gerontology

There are at least three parallels between the emergence of critical gerontology and the development of feminist theory-building in various academic disciplines. First, reverberations from the Frankfurt School can be found in the ageing literature in the 1930s. Second, just as there is no single brand of feminism, so too there are variegated strands of critical gerontology, which reflect both the diversity of the aged population and the multifaceted nature of gerontologic inquiry. Third, critical gerontology has greater impact when linked to 'mainstream' ideas when it is viewed as an exotic supplement to ongoing research. Let us consider each parallel in turn.

Philosophers, scientists, theologians, political economists, novelists and artists have been reflecting on the meanings and experiences of growing older since ancient times. Medieval treatises on longevity contain helpful hints for health that remain useful today. Only in the twentieth century, however, did 'gerontology' become a collective intellectual enterprise that sought to mobilize the theories and methods of experts from a variety of disciplines and professions to deal with the *problem* of old age. Differences between G. Stanley Hall's *Senescence* (1922) and Edmund V. Cowdry's *Problems of Aging* (1939) illustrate the abrupt shift that occurred. Hall's compendium of insights from religion, philosophy, history as well as the basic sciences aimed to prove that 'intelligent and well-conserved senectitude has very important social and anthropological functions in the world, not hitherto utilized or even recognized' (Hall 1922: v; see also Cole 1992). The psychologist intended to revise conventional wisdom, as he had done in *Adolescence*, by swaying a mass audience, not experts. Fifteen years later, Cowdry gathered more than two dozen of the best scientists in the USA together to Woods Hole, Massachusetts, to set out the parameters for a new field of research. His collection was a 'handbook', authoritative because it appeared both exhaustive and scientific (Achenbaum 1989).

Introducing the highly specialized chapters, ranging from 'Senescence and death in protozoa and invertebrates' to 'Skeleton, locomotor system and teeth', were chapters by Lawrence K. Frank, an intellectual gadfly and foundation officer, and John Dewey, arguably the era's most famous North American philosopher. Frank urged researchers to ask big questions to clarify 'the concept of the psychosomatic unity of the organism' (Frank 1939: xv). He noted that 'in all studies of growth and of ageing, time is of the greatest significance' (p. xvii). Dewey went even further than Frank in stressing the need for multidisciplinary approaches to comprehending the problems of ageing:

> It is my conviction that the many perplexing problems now attendant upon human old age have a psychological-social origin . . . Biological processes are at the roots of the problems and of the methods of solving them, but the biological processes take place in economic, political and cultural contexts. They are inextricably woven with these contexts so that one reacts upon the other in all sorts of intricate ways. We need to know the ways in which social contexts react back into biological processes as well as to know the ways in which the biological processes condition life.
>
> (Dewey 1939: xxvi)

No recent spokesperson for critical gerontology has framed the 'problem' better than this. Dewey grasped that problems were socially constructed; growth and ageing occurred in fluid, often contradictory, contexts. A penetrating, reflexive scrutiny of assumptions and phenomena was critical: 'Science and philosophy meet on common ground in their joint interest in discovering the processes of normal growth and in the institution of conditions which will favor and support ever continued growth' (Dewey 1939: xxvii).

A new cohort of philosophers and historians urges researchers on ageing to challenge their own assumptions about their work. In *What Does It Mean to Grow Old?*, Thomas R. Cole and Sally Gadow 'shifted attention from the "human values" approach that informed earlier work in humanistic gerontology toward issues of personal, textual, historical, and cultural meaning' (Cole and Gadow 1986; quotation from Cole 1993: viii). According to philosopher H.R. Moody, the humanities must challenge positivism by assaulting instrumentalism. Moody also anticipates a second parallel between critical gerontology and feminist theory by stressing the diversity inherent in both. Some critical gerontology, contends Moody, deals mainly with fundamental epistemological issues. Others represent themselves as political gerontology and humanistic gerontology (Moody 1988, 1993).

Experts from the humanities are not alone in the struggle. Several prominent researchers on ageing, trained in the social sciences, advocate critical gerontology. Two examples may suffice. Educational psychologist Dale Dannefer charges that 'the neglect of heterogeneity was proposed not to be an isolated anomaly, but the product of the systematic logical tendencies deriving from the language and paradigmatic assumptions guiding research on age – in other words from the particular names given by social science to the phenomena it studies' (Dannefer 1988: 373). Research on ageing must transcend its current scientistic assumptions. In similar fashion, political gerontologists have bemoaned social contradictions that inhere in policy-making by applying their theory to practice. 'Consistent with the goal of Critical Theory,' argues Carroll Estes (1991: 344), 'the project must inevitably engage in action. It requires moving beyond positivist assumptions . . . to critically examine the social and cultural production of aging and gerontological knowledge at their base and to attend to the class, generational, gender, and racial/ethnic divisions and ideological forces embedded in their production and reproduction.' Among other things, Estes and her colleagues have excoriated the *bio-medicalization* of ageing, whose 'extension to and control over all aspects of life not only diminish its own effectiveness, but inhibit society from understanding and addressing complex issues in the appropriate and innovative ways necessary' (Estes and Binney 1989: 596).

Estes over time has become more 'radical', not only politically but in her citations: she draws heavily from neo-Marxist political economists and sociologists in Britain and the European continent. This penchant for *inter*disciplinary theory building goes far beyond now familiar claims for gerontological multidisciplinarity. At best, there is usually an exchange of ideas by researchers from different disciplines. Critical theory, however, tends to facilitate the weaving together of disparate intellectual ideas into a powerful critique of prevailing gerontological ideas (Achenbaum 1995). The result is particularly striking in the work of anthropologists Andrea Sankar and Mark Luborsky, who seek to extend the perspectives of critical gerontology by applying a 'critical gaze' to the cultural dimensions of ageing: 'An appreciation of the structuring role of culture can lead us to a more accurate depiction of the reality we study as well as a profound appreciation for the challenges involved in the creation and implementation of effective policy'[1] (Sankar 1993: 438; see also Luborsky and Sankar 1993).

Despite these similarities, three differences between critical gerontology and feminist theory-building must be acknowledged. First, researchers on ageing who put 'critical theory' into gerontology tend to be peripheral. Newcomers, such as experts in the humanities, are expected to fit into existing structures, not create organizations of their own. Bench scientists resist radical alternatives more than other scholars. 'Evolutionary gerontology should strictly avoid taking on the imperatives of critical gerontology, and critical gerontologists should take pains not to develop "evolutionary ethics" concerning the treatment of the elderly,' argues Michael Rose (1993: 73). 'One might imagine some kind of ageist ideology coming out of a marriage between critical gerontology and evolutionary gerontology, an ideology that might advocate the compulsory euthanasia of the retired on the grounds of their evolutionary unimportance.' So while 'feminist' and even 'queer' theory commands attention in the humanities and social sciences, critical gerontology does not.

Specialization works against critical theory's integrative possibilities. Gerontology, contends James Birren, is 'a land of many islands of data with few bridges between them' (Birren 1989: 144). The field remains, as Leonard Cain described in 1964, a 'new and burgeoning field [that] represents a peculiar amalgam of scientific research and reformist commitment with the attributes of a major social movement' (Cain 1964: 459). These characterizations suggest a second reason why it has been so difficult to integrate critical gerontology into research and practice dominated by big science. Intellectually, conflict is best expressed among disciplinary peers. Politically, most gerontologists conform to the principles and strategies of interest-group liberalism. In this milieu, even those who advance critical theory tend to treat aspects of parts of the ageing enterprise as if they constituted gerontology's entire domain. Risk-taking is selective, and usually discipline-driven.

Finally (and here I speculate), academics generally deplore sexism, but they repress their ageism. 'The conventional psychology of aging is almost completely devoted to the study of its discontents: aging as depletion, aging as catastrophe, aging as mortality,' observes David Gutmann (1987: 5). 'At best the aged are deemed barely capable of staving off disaster, but they are certainly not deemed capable of developing new capacities or of seeking out new challenges by their own choice (and even for the sheer hell of it).' Reflecting the views of the dominant culture, scholars like to view ageing as something that happens to others. This perspective has been deflated most recently by Betty Friedan, who makes an analogy between raising women's consciousness and discovering 'the Fountain of Age'. None the less, discerning women of all ages can perceive the power of feminism; few researchers of age have lived long enough to appreciate the wisdom that comes in part through acknowledging the finitude of life (Friedan 1993: 620). To many gerontologists, who fear their own obsolescence, staying productive bespeaks successful ageing. Too few of our successful elders – Wilma Donahue, Bernice Neugarten and Matilda White Riley are exceptions – have offered introspective commentaries on their lives' careers (Riley 1988; Donahue 1991). Consequently, young gerontologists rarely get 'inside' the experiences of ageing. Lacking the requisite balance between introspective detachment and passionate commitment, they fail 'in measure in rescuing age from the scandalous contempt in which it is held' (Woodward 1991: 193).

## Invigorating critical gerontology with feminist theory

More than was true of the Frankfurt School, most theory-builders nowadays acknowledge the limitations and possibilities of working in a particular historical and ideological milieu. 'Interest has been shifted from truth to relevance, and from description to critique' (Bal 1990: 133). Critical theory enables scholars to amalgamate disparate ideas from Marxism, psychoanalysis and deconstructionism. It is a device for breaking disciplinary boundaries and investigating broader opportunities. Yet in other domains critical theory produces paradoxical results. Feminism has altered existing academic structures, encouraging a greater plurality of practices, without radically transforming them (Klein 1993). It has not yet closed the gap in many fields, including gerontology, between abstract theory and existing disciplinary arrangements.

That said, critical gerontology would benefit from an infusion of feminism. Differences in life expectancy, the feminization of poverty and the psychology of ageing all demand greater attention to the gender-specific dimensions of late life. Additive and reflexive, feminist theory already intersects with much gerontologic theory. Self-reflexive blending of perspectives will sharpen ageing issues. 'Disciplining is practiced by reproducing boundaries: feminist practices transgress boundaries and generate new visions – from the margins where boundaries are inherently conspicuous' (Peterson 1993: 260).

# Note

1 Thus it is not by accident that Sankar (1991) subtitled her *Dying at Home* a guide for family caregivers.

# References

Achenbaum, W.A. (1989) One United States approach to gerontological theory building. *Ageing and Society*, 9, 179–88.

Achembaum, W.A. (1995) *Crossing Frontiers*. New York: Cambridge University Press.

Bal, M. (1990) Visual poetics, in M. Kreiswirth and M.A. Cheetham (eds) *Theory between the Disciplines*. Ann Arbor: University of Michigan Press.

Baym, N. (1992) *Feminism and American Literary History*. New Brunswick, NJ: Rutgers University.

Bernard, J. (1973) My four revolutions, *American Journal of Sociology*, 78, 773–91.

Birren, J. (1989) My perspective on research on aging, in V.L. Bengtson and K.W. Schaie (eds) *The Course of Later Life*. New York: Springer.

Butterfield, L.H., Friedlander, M. and Kline, M.J. (eds) (1975) *The Book of Abigail and John*. Cambridge, MA: Harvard University Press.

Cain, L.D. (1964) Review, *American Sociological Review*, 29, 459.

Cole, T. (1992) *Journey of Life*. New York: Cambridge University Press.

Cole, T. (1993) Preface, in T. Cole, A. Achenbaum, P. Jakobi and R. Kastenbaum (eds) *Voices and Visions of Aging*. New York: Springer.

Cole, T. and Gadow, S. (1986) *What Does It Mean to Grow Old? Reflections from the Humanities*. Durham, NC: Duke University Press.

Costello, C. and Stone, A.J. (eds) (1994) *The American Woman*. New York: W.W. Norton.

Cott, N.F. (1977) *The Bonds of Womanhood*. New Haven, CT: Yale University Press.

Cott, N.F. and Pleck, E.H. (eds) (1979) *A Heritage of Her Own*. New York: Simon and Schuster.

Cowdry, E.V. (1939) *Problems of Aging*. Baltimore: Williams and Wilkins.

Dannefer, D. (1988) Neglect of variability in the study of aging, in J.E. Birren and V.L. Bengtson (eds) *Emergent Theories of Aging*. New York: Springer.

Davidson, N. (1988) *The Failure of Feminism*. Buffalo, NY: Prometheus Books.

Dewey, J. (1939) Introduction, in E.V. Cowdry (ed.) *Problems of Aging*. Baltimore: Williams and Wilkins.

Donahue, W.T. (1991) A survivor's career, in F.M. Carp (ed.) *Lives of Career Women*. New York: Plenum, 23–41.

Estes, C.L. (1991) Epilogue, in M. Minkler and C.L. Estes (eds) *Critical Perspectives on Aging: the Political and Moral Economy of Growing Old*. Amityville, NY: Baywood Publishing.

Estes, C.L. and Binney, E.A. (1989) The biomedicalization of aging: dangers and dilemmas, *The Gerontologist*, 29, 596.

Fine, M. (ed.) (1992) *Disruptive Voices*. Ann Arbor: University of Michigan Press.

Fine, M. and Gordon, S.M. (1992) Feminist transformations of/despite psychology, in M. Fine (ed.) *Disruptive Voices*. Ann Arbor: University of Michigan Press.

Frank, L.F. (1939) Foreword, in E.V. Cowdry (ed.) *Problems of Ageing*. Baltimore: Williams and Wilkins.

Fraser, N. and Nicholson, L.J. (1990) Social criticism without philosophy, in L.J. Nicholson (ed.) *Feminism/Postmodernism*. New York: Routledge.

Friedan, B. (1963) *The Feminine Mystique*. New York: Dell.

Friedan, B. (1993) *The Fountain of Age*. New York: Simon and Schuster.

Glieck, J. (1987) *Chaos*. New York: Penguin.

Gutmann, D. (1987) *Reclaimed Powers*. New York: Basic Books.

Hall, G.S. (1922) *Senescence*. New York: D. Appleton.

Harding, S. (1987) *Feminism and Methodology: Social Science Issues*. Bloomington: Indiana University Press.

Honneth, A. (1987) Critical theory, in A. Giddens and J.H. Turner (eds) *Social Theory Today*. Stanford, CA: Stanford University Press.

Keller, E.F. (1982) Feminism and science, *Signs: Journal of Women in Culture and Society*, 7(3), 589–602.

Klein, J.T. (1993) Blurring, cracking and crossing: permeation and the fracturing of discipline, in E. Messer-Davidow, D.R. Shumway and D.J. Sylvan (eds) *Knowledges*. Charlottesville, University of Virginia Press, 193–4.

Krieswirth, M. and Cheetham, M.A. (eds) (1990) *Theory between the Disciplines*. Ann Arbor: University of Michigan Press.

Luborsky, M.R. and Sankar, A. (1993) Extending the critical gerontology perspective: cultural dimensions, *The Gerontologist*, 33, 440–3.

Moody, H.R. (1988) Toward a critical gerontology: the contribution of the humanities to the theory of aging, in J.E. Birren and V.L. Bengtson (eds) *Emergent Theories of Aging*. New York: Springer.

Moody, H.R. (1993) Overview: what is critical gerontology and why is it important?, in T. Cole, A. Achenbaum, P. Jakobi and R. Kastenbaum (eds) *Voices and Visions of Aging*. New York: Springer.

Morantz-Sanchez, R.M. (1985) *Sympathy and Science*. New York: Oxford University Press.

Nicholson, L.J. (1990) *Feminism/Postmodernism*. New York: Routledge.

Peterson, V.S. (1993) *Disciplining practiced/practices*: gendered states and politics, in E. Messer-Davidow, D.R. Shumway and D.J. Sylvan (eds) *Knowledges*. Charlottesville, University of Virginia Press, 193–4.

Riley, M.W. (ed.) (1988) *Sociological Lives*. Newbury Park, CA: Sage.

Rose, M. (1993) Evolutionary gerontology and critical gerontology: let's just be friends, in T. Cole, A. Achenbaum, P. Jakobi and R. Kastenbaum (eds) *Voices and Visions of Aging*. New York: Springer.

Rosenburg, R. (1983) *Beyond Separate Spheres*. New Haven, CT: Yale University Press.

Salzman, J. (ed.) (1986) *The Cambridge Handbook of American Literature*. New York: Cambridge University Press.

Sankar, A. (1991) *Dying at Home: a Guide for Family Caregivers*. Baltimore: Johns Hopkins University Press.

Sankar, A. (1993) Culture, research and policy, *The Gerontologist*, 33, 438.

Stacey, J. and Thorne, B. (1993) The missing feminist revolution in sociology, in L.S. Kauffman (ed.) *American Feminist Thought at Century's End*. Cambridge, MA: Blackwell.

Stanley, L. and Wise, S. (1993) *Breaking out Again: Feminist Ontology and Epistemology*. London: RKP (new edition).

Woloch, N. (1991) Education, in E. Foner and J.A. Garraty (eds) *The Readers' Companion to American History*. Boston: Houghton Mifflin.

Woodward, K. (1991) *Aging and Its Discontents*. Bloomington: Indiana University Press.

Ziman, J. (1994) *Prometheus Bound*. New York: Cambridge University Press.

## 3 KEN BLAKEMORE

# From minorities to majorities: perspectives on culture, ethnicity and ageing in British gerontology

The primary purpose of this chapter is not to provide a comprehensive review of current literature on ageing and ethnicity. Nor is it to discuss a particular hypothesis or piece of research in detail. It is to prompt some critical thoughts about the 'culture-blind' assumptions which underpin much social gerontology, and about the relative neglect of cross-cultural and comparative perspectives.

As a guide to contemporary gerontology, this chapter reviews a selection of articles published in the journal *Ageing and Society* from 1981 to 1994. A more specialized journal, such as *Cross-Cultural Gerontology*, would, of course, reveal a wider range of both cross-national comparative work and attention to contrasts between minority and majority patterns of ageing within countries. However, *Ageing and Society* is the flagship of 'mainstream' British gerontology. Its publications represent the priorities and interests evident in the field.

Hardly an issue of *Ageing and Society* has gone by without at least two articles from outside the United Kingdom. Therefore, this chapter is not a criticism of a lack of international perspectives in British gerontology or of uninterest in national differences in patterns of ageing. But it is easy to assume that either other-national or cross-national studies amount to cross-*cultural* studies, when mostly they are not. Considerations of culture and ethnicity are often minimal or non-existent in single nation or cross-national studies (as examples, see Nies *et al.* 1991; Harper 1992).

This is not to undervalue the contribution of such national or regional case studies, each of which adds awareness of the rich variety of patterns of ageing and of the social, economic and political influences upon the role and position of older people in different countries. However, in a decade of contributions to *Ageing and Society* only a handful of articles *explicitly* discuss questions of culture or ethnicity, or draw comparisons between different ethnic groups. On the other hand, others *inexplicitly* deal with such questions, and some examples will be mentioned below.

*Ageing and Society*, comprehensive and international in focus though it is, offers only one indicator of the state of the art. However, other indicators, such as key texts in social gerontology (for example, Victor 1987; Fennell *et al.* 1988; Arber and Evandrou 1993), show broadly the same picture. There is much attention in British social gerontology to questions of social class, gender and other kinds of differentiation. Culture and ethnicity, on the other hand, while receiving some attention in some of the texts, are always bracketed off in distinct sections or chapters rather than being integrated into the whole.

## Do culture and ethnicity matter?

In making these points, I am not suggesting that questions of ethnicity and culture are always of supreme or even of considerable importance for understanding ageing. Setting aside for a moment the difficult question of what culture, ethnicity and ethnic relations are (Brah 1994), there are many instances in which the ethnic identities of older people have little or no bearing on outcomes. Other influences – economic, political or historical – may be much more important in shaping either the ageing process or the social policies which affect older people.

The point is rather that in Britain, as in other countries where minority ethnic communities are marginalized and form less than 10 per cent of the population, social gerontology has failed to consider ethnic and cultural influences where these *do* count.

Cultural and ethnic factors can have a highly significant influence on both the experience of ageing and policy-makers' perceptions of what older people need. To give one example, Jylha and Jokela's (1990) comparison of loneliness in older people in Greece and Finland illustrates how significant the cultural context may be in predisposing people to feel lonely or to perceive loneliness. They report the interesting but not unique finding that loneliness can be more evident in communities where few old people live alone and where cultural values of familial support are still relatively strong but undergoing rapid change (as in Greece). Paradoxically, in communities where much higher proportions live alone (as in Finland), loneliness can be perceived as a problem less often. These findings parallel those of cross-ethnic studies elsewhere, such as in the United States (Cantor 1976) and Britain (Blakemore and Boneham 1994: 54).

Cultural and ethnic perspectives could make contributions to gerontological theory as well as to policy-relevant issues such as perceptions of loneliness and changing patterns of family support. For example, how far do feminist perspectives on later life need to be modified in the light of cultural and ethnic differences in gender roles? Are the effects of post-industrial capitalism upon later life, as portrayed by political economy and structured dependency theories, mitigated by the protective role of certain ethnic communities, for example, by providing older people with respected and valued roles? And how are the ideas underlying activity theory, role theory or theories of disengagement to be recast to take account of ethnic heterogeneity?

These questions, which hint at the potential for a considerable enrichment of gerontology by the inclusion of ethnic and cultural perspectives, lead to another question: why, if they are so important, have ethnic and cultural aspects of ageing been neglected in Britain?

First, there is an understandable concern in the social sciences that apparent reliance on 'culturalist' explanations can problematize or pathologize minority groups. Earlier studies of culture and ethnicity often appeared to neglect the realities of racism and of unequal power relations between black minorities and a white majority because they tended to focus on minority ways of life in isolation from wider power structures.

Thus, among those concerned with race relations today, any reference to 'culture' as a primary or even conditioning influence would almost certainly be met with sharp criticism. To a degree, these reactions are justified. However, as Holzberg (1982) argues, when the legitimacy of *any* discussion of the effects of ethnicity and culture on ageing was rejected, the baby was thrown out with the bath water. Reductionist accounts which place all the emphasis on culture are of course misleading. But by the same token, accounts of ageing which explain away or disregard substantial cultural differences by reference to the 'realities' of class, patriarchy, economics and so on are equally reductionist.

The dangers of the culture-blind approach, identified by Holzberg, are mirrored in Brah's unease about the 'ascendancy of Marxist thought in British academia during the 1970s and early 1980s', which, while it seemed to try to avoid reductionism,

> ended up reproducing a framework which emphasised the primacy of class. For a period such class reductionism inhibited analyses between the relationship between class, racism, gender, sexuality, or other markers of social differentiation. It undermined attempts to analyse issues of culture, ethnicity and identity.
>
> (Brah 1994: 811)

## Applying culture and ethnicity to 'majority' ageing

Given the highly charged nature of debates about race and ethnicity, perhaps it was not surprising that many scholars, not only those in gerontology, steered clear of the race relations minefield. In Britain, culture and ethnicity have been racialized and are usually assumed to be terms applicable only to black minorities.

Thus, in most studies of ageing, the ethnic identities of white people are taken for granted or simply disregarded, whether they are in the majority community or in white minorities such as the Irish, Jewish or Polish communities. Misleading generalizations such as 'black culture' and 'white culture' cement the racialized view of ethnicity and culture.

White scholars may feel reluctant to involve themselves in a field in which they feel unqualified to speak or to conduct research. This is a perception which 'radical' researchers and 'anti-racist' trainers (both black and white), particularly in the field of social work, are only too happy to encourage.

The neglect of cultural and ethnic dimensions of ageing is particularly unfortunate because, far from masking the realities of power, they can pinpoint key determinants of power and status and the conflicts that may arise between ethnic communities. In Northern Ireland, for instance, it would be interesting to find out how far older people act as repositories of communal distinctiveness and division, acting (if they have any influence) to maintain and redraw boundaries between Catholics and Protestants, or how far older members of churches, political groups and other organizations tend to build bridges or reinterpret cultural or religious divisions in ways that minimize overt conflict.

Lest readers are sidetracked into deeper thoughts about the Northern Ireland case, however, it is important to stress that this is but one example of many cases of cultural or ethnic difference, and of relationships between minorities and majorities which range from highly equal to unequal. The point of the Northern Irish case is simply to underline how reference to culture and ethnicity should prompt discussion of power and the politicization of ethnic differences rather than obscure such discussion.

In sum, *culture* can be taken to embrace all the things that distinguish a way of life: its social institutions (for example, family structures), religious beliefs and values, and preferences in terms of social behaviour, diet and dress.

*Ethnicity* is a concept which includes culture, and often the two terms can be used interchangeably; for instance, we may refer to the Irish or Italian communities in Britain as minority cultural or ethnic groups. However, ethnicity in addition implies a *political* identity. Ethnic groups can only be understood by reference to ethnic *relations*, or the relationships between identified groups, and these inevitably have dimensions of power and status. Thus, as with racial identity, ethnicity cannot exist in a vacuum and can only be brought about through social and political interaction and a process of social construction.

Often, leaders of minority communities engineer a common ethnic identity for the purposes of political mobilization or in order to lobby central and local government for resources. The emergence of an 'Afro-Caribbean' community in Britain is a good example of the creation of a single ethnic identity from a multiplicity of competing identities.

Thus, as Barth's influential (1969) work on ethnicity suggested, ethnic boundaries and relationships, whether conflictual or otherwise, are as important in defining ethnic identity as are the 'internal' or cultural characteristics of one's group. Ethnic identity is not simply a matter of how *we* define ourselves in relation to other groups, but also depends upon the degree of power *other* groups can mobilize to establish their definitions of us.

These insights show how we may move from specific examples of cultural and ethnic difference such as Northern Ireland to a wide variety of situations in which older people find themselves. Three examples follow.

First, the growing trend towards migration in later life (for instance, English-speaking people settling in north Wales, or in southern Spain) is leading to increasing cultural diversity in some regions, with implications for the need to negotiate new ethnic boundaries which are complicated by divisions of age.

Less obvious, but no less important, are the differences which arise from the relationship between class and culture (or class subcultures) in British society. Here, different subgroups belong to the same overarching 'ethnic' group (for example, white English people), but people are often sharply aware of differences in values, manners, diet and accent. These class and/or regional differences can be extremely important in older people's judgements of all kinds of social provisions, including the quality or acceptability of institutional care settings, or of sheltered housing schemes (as an example of a discussion which expresses feelings about class and cultural preferences, see Jefferys 1996).

In drawing contrasts between ethnic minorities and the majority, it is all too easy to assume that the latter are culturally homogeneous. Yet, as distinctions of class culture show, the white majority is far from being a culturally homogeneous whole. Cultural differences play a highly significant role in explaining variations in attitudes to health and independence in later life, the ways in which pain or discomfort are expressed, or the expectations different groups have of the roles of sons, daughters and other family members in providing care or support for older relatives.

Finally, there is the possibility that older people, as a growing minority in an increasingly age-categorized society, will form their own subculture (Rose 1965). As Markides and Mindel (1987: 27–8) suggest, though, it seems unlikely that a homogeneous age-based culture will develop very far beyond the sharing of certain cultural products or styles. As with youth subcultures, pre-existing class and income, gender and ethnic differences among older people will prevent the development of a common subculture of later life.

However, if adapted to take account of diversity, and if combined with biographical and oral history perspectives on ageing, the basic idea of cohort-related subcultural groups has gained acceptance in social gerontology. For example, we may identify 'women who received higher education in the 1960s' to discuss whether they form a distinctive cohort: whether, for example, their particular conjunction of biography and cultural experiences will result in their becoming a distinctively different group when they begin to reach pensionable age from 2002 onwards.

The point about these three examples is not that they are unheard of in gerontology, nor that they are entirely absent from the pages of journals such as *Ageing and Society*, but rather that research at the interface between ethnicity, cultural difference and ageing has been relatively neglected.

However, there is a body of work which is sensitive to these questions, to a greater or lesser degree. The remainder of the chapter identifies two models, or a framework for understanding this work, in order to promote discussion of 'where we go from here'. It is followed by a conclusion which discusses possibilities for future research, including comparisons between minority and majority ageing.

|  | Research *inexplicitly* dealing with cultural aspects of ageing; culture/ethnicity unstated or part of the background | Research *explicitly* evaluating or discussing cultural aspects |
|---|---|---|
| Comparative or cross-cultural studies | (a) | (b) |
| Single nation or single community/ case study | (c) | (d) |

*Figure 3.1*

## Models of 'culture-sensitive' gerontology

In order to take stock of research already completed on cultural and ethnic themes, it might be helpful to think of a basic distinction between 'explicit' and 'inexplicit' studies, on the one hand, and of 'comparative' and 'non-comparative' studies on the other (see Figure 3.1).

### Inexplicit studies

These studies do not make any explicit references to, or observations about, culture or ethnicity, beyond perhaps identifying who the groups are, where respondents live and so on. Such work may be comparative in nature (a in Figure 3.1), but it is not explicitly cross-*cultural* research. As stated at the outset, this is not a comment on the value of such research. Questions of ethnicity and culture may not be relevant, or simply are not a feature of the researcher's hypothesis. Some studies aim to reach conclusions about the politics or economics of policies affecting older people, rather than focusing on subjects which are more readily associated with cultural or ethnic factors, such as family structures and family change, or subjective and psychological aspects of ageing.

However, it is up to the reader to work out what the effects upon findings might be of the largely unstated cultural backgrounds of respondents, or the cultural and ethnic mix of the countries in which research has been conducted. Moreover, we are usually left to draw our own conclusions about the ways in which results gathered in one cultural setting would compare with results of similar studies in other settings.

Examples published in *Ageing and Society* from outside Britain are Bonanno and Calasanti's (1986) research on the political economy of old age in southern Italy, Checkoway and Morales-Martinez (1990) on health promotion in Costa Rica and Hampson (1985) on social welfare in Zimbabwe.

Other studies *have* explored questions which are quite specifically cultural or ethnic, but the researchers' conclusions do not explicitly discuss the characteristics of the society or culture under study. Examples are Chetkow-Yanoov's (1986) research on leadership among Israeli professionals, Chappell and Marshall (1992) on social integration and care-giving in Bermuda, Moller (1994) on inter-generational relationships in South Africa and Synak (1987) on ageing in Poland.

However, there are differences among these non-comparative, inexplicit studies in the degree to which ethnic and cultural factors are downplayed or ignored. For example, it is only in passing that we learn from Moller's paper that this is a study of a black (mainly Zulu) community in a specific area, and one is left wondering how far Moller's findings on the effects of political violence would be replicated among other ethnic groups.

Chappell and Marshall, on the other hand, are very concerned to illustrate the distinctiveness of Bermudan society, which apparently has exceptionally strong levels of informal community support of older people compared with Western industrialized societies. However, the causes of this distinctiveness are not explored, beyond Bermuda's being a small-scale society. One is again left wondering how Bermuda compares with other, similar examples. In Jamaica, for example, respect for and support of older people is conditional upon their economic and social status (Foner 1973, 1979).

Inexplicitness in approaches to cultural and ethnic aspects of ageing is also apparent in British-based research: for example, that of Cunningham-Burley (1986), Harper (1987), Jerrome (1981) and Wenger (1982, 1985).

Cunningham-Burley's paper is of grandparenthood among a small sample of 'ordinary' grandparents in Scotland. But in this otherwise valuable study, the impact of Scottish identity or of regional and cultural influences on expectations of family life and the grandparent role are not explicitly discussed. Similarly, Jerrome (1981) discusses 'broadly middle class' women, but their Englishness is assumed rather than explored as a source of constraints and opportunities in making friends. What would a Japanese or North American gerontologist make of Jerrome's findings on the nature of friendship in English culture?

Looked at the other way – that is, from a British perspective – Matthews's (1983) paper on friendship among 30 men and 30 women in the USA mentions 'diverse backgrounds', but little or nothing about how the cultural aspects of these backgrounds affect notions of friendship; consequently it is harder for the British reader to find points of comparison.

Wenger's research is perhaps the closest, in the 'inexplicit' category, to an explicit recognition of cultural or ethnic influences on family ties and community integration (in north Wales). There are frequent references to the characteristics of local towns and villages, and to the significance of the Welsh language. Wenger and colleagues also make many comparative references, so that her work falls into both the a and b categories of Figure 3.1. However, this is not research which explicitly seeks to explore the impact of the Welsh context or Welsh culture on the quality of supportive relationships. Rather, the emphasis is more upon the ways in which demographic factors affect levels of community support: for instance, the rates of in-migration and out-migration, population stability and density.

*Explicit studies*

A survey of *Ageing and Society* from 1981 to 1994 reveals a much smaller group of articles which fall into the explicit categories b and d: among 11 examples there are, for example, papers by Bowling and Farquar (1993), Hazan (1984), Mays (1983) and Starrett *et al.* (1987).

To reiterate a point, the fact that these are explicitly studies of culture or ethnicity is not a comment on the quality or value of the research itself, as compared with the 'inexplicit' studies mentioned above. It is only to suggest that, from the point of view of cultural aspects of ageing, this kind of work facilitates comparison and helps the reader to contextualize results.

Bowling and Farquar's (1993) study of perceptions of health among older Jewish people in London, for example, not only discusses responses in the sample but also draws attention to other studies of the relationship between ethnicity and perceptions of health, illness and pain.

Mays (1983) and Starrett *et al.* (1987) also discuss health and well-being, but mainly in terms of health and social service utilization. Mays refers to research on Asian minority communities in the United Kingdom, and Starrett *et al.* to Puerto Rican older people in the United States. Both explicitly compare minority with majority patterns of service use, exploring cultural and ethnic factors as explanations for differences.

However, some of the research explicitly concerned with culture and ethnicity is not comparative and falls into the d category (see above). Hazan's (1984) discussion of the 'time universe' of older Jewish people fits this category, as does Davis's (1985) study of conflict among octogenarians in an American community and Reid's (1985) discussion of the status of older Aboriginal people in Australia. Each of these studies is an in-depth examination of a particular community or cultural group. But by integrating wider theoretical perspectives into their work – for example, in terms of the role of religious symbolism in structuring the everyday world of older people – these studies make it possible to consider implications for other research on cultural aspects of ageing.

## Conclusion: towards multicultural gerontology?

As this brief survey of gerontological priorities has shown, work on cultural and ethnic aspects of ageing is as yet in its infancy in the United Kingdom, especially when compared with the amount of attention given to ethnic and racial issues in other multicultural societies, such as the United States and Australia.

Where gerontological research has explicitly explored questions of culture and ethnicity, the focus has been more upon the former than the latter. In other words, the majority of examples from *Ageing and Society* mentioned above are easily bracketed under the heading 'cultural aspects of ageing'. Common concerns among researchers have been the connections between culture and the subjective experience of illness and ageing, or between culture and perceptions of friendship, kinship and other sources of support. Much less common is an interest in relations between ethnic groups or in the power dimension of relationships between older people of different ethnic backgrounds, or between older people of one ethnic/racial background and younger people of another.

What paths could British gerontology take towards greater recognition not only of the influence of cultural factors on ageing in the majority population but also of the significance of ethnic boundaries and divisions and the power inequalities attendant upon these?

### Inter-ethnic relations and age

One path lies in the direction of exploring the significance of cultural and ethnic difference in the relationships older people have with those who have more power than they do, and whose decisions can profoundly affect their lives. Examples that spring to mind are doctor–patient relationships, or relationships between older people and care workers or other social service practitioners. If, for instance, the client or patient belongs to a minority community and the professional or care worker to the majority, there is the possibility that minority status may jeopardize chances of being treated sensitively or of being heard with respect: a language difference and the professional's stereotypical views of the minority community may play a large part in this.

On the other hand, not much thought has been given to situations in which the older person from the majority white community is dealt with by a professional or carer from a minority community – for instance, a doctor of Indian descent or an Afro-Caribbean nurse or home care worker – yet in certain parts of the United Kingdom this is an increasingly likely possibility. What kinds of ethnic stereotyping fly back and forth in such encounters, and – if they surface – how do they affect treatment or care plans, and the eventual outcomes for the older people concerned?

Lest the latter examples suggest a 'racial' as much as an 'ethnic' difference in encounters, we should remind ourselves that the ethnic dimension in relationships between older and younger people of the *same* 'race' is a neglected field of research: the experiences of Irish people in Britain, for instance, are particularly under-researched in both welfare studies and social gerontology. Given the ambivalent nature of relations between the Irish and English communities, studies of ageing among Irish migrants to Britain would offer an excellent opportunity to begin to disentangle the respective influences upon the ageing process of ethnicity, with its connotations of power and status, as well as of social class and other factors.

### The lessons of minority ageing

Another path for multicultural gerontology may be found through beginning to apply what we are learning about minority ageing to the majority. As a 'minority in a minority', Asian, black and possibly some white minority ethnic elderly people have experiences which offer ways of assessing the relative influences of age *vis-à-vis* other influences on the income, status, power, health and well-being of older people.

If there is a gulf between 'majority' older people and at least some older people from minority communities, in terms of either objectively measured living standards or subjective aspects of well-being, this would suggest that age and age discrimination are relatively weak influences on the position and welfare of older people. On the other hand, declining minority–majority differences would seem to indicate that factors specific to each community (including ethnic and cultural factors), or ethnic and racial discrimination, are less powerful influences than the overarching effects of age and ageing – whether these are primarily biological or social, or a mixture of both.

These points about minority–majority comparisons have been made elsewhere (Dowd and Bengtson 1978; Blakemore and Boneham 1994). However, it is worth restating that although there is now a substantial amount of research on ageing in Britain's minority ethnic groups, very little research has yet to be completed on systematic comparisons between majority and minority ethnic groups. Similarly, little has been done to apply 'mainstream' theories of ageing (for instance, biological theories of ageing and predictors of longevity, or political economy approaches and theories of structured dependency) to minority and majority samples in the same study.

### Comparative studies of migration and ageing

A third path for British gerontology to follow, in order to address neglected questions of ethnicity and ethnic relations, would be to compare the migration experiences of older people in the majority community (including migration in later life or at an earlier point in the life course) with experiences of international migration, especially among those in minority communities. Long-distance migration, whether international or within Britain, and whether forced or voluntary, has become an increasingly common feature of the life histories of older people and, given the economic, political and demographic upheavals of the late twentieth century, will result in a much more diverse and heterogeneous population of older people in the future.

Yet migration is as neglected a field of social gerontology as the study of cultural and ethnic aspects of ageing. This is surprising, given the scientific possibilities offered by the comparison of migrant and non-migrant older people; for instance, in terms of biological theories of ageing, one important question is whether, or how far, migration impairs health or shortens lives, or whether it is always the case that the initial health status of long-distance migrants, a self-selected group, cancels out the effects of any 'migration stress'. Moreover, do political and economic factors, including elements of protectiveness and support when successful members of minority communities provide support and care facilities for older people, mitigate any adverse effects from migration?

Finally, the main argument of this chapter has not been that every aspect of gerontology or every research project should be permeated with questions of culture, ethnicity, migration or comparisons between minority and majority groups. There are substantial areas in which these questions are irrelevant. But there is some research which already contains promising avenues for further development of cultural and ethnic questions: the 'inexplicit' studies. It is as if they had been 'wired' for ethnic or cultural comparisons to be made, but there are no connections or sockets for readers to plug into. In most cases, only a few explicit references to what makes the group culturally distinctive, and how cultural factors may affect the hypothesis, are needed to facilitate comparison. With greater attention to comparative observation, therefore, the outlook for a more multicultural and less Anglo-centric gerontology is encouraging.

Less encouraging, though, if the pages of *Ageing and Society* are taken as a reasonably accurate representation of British gerontology over the past 15 years, is the impression that little or nothing has been done to integrate or compare research findings on minority communities with those on the majority. 'Ethnicity' has too often been thought of as 'something to do with minorities in the inner city', and it is high time that such ghettoized thinking was challenged.

## References

Arber, S. and Evandrou, M. (1993) *Ageing, Independence and the Life Course*. London: Jessica Kingsley Publishers.

Barth, F. (1969) *Ethnic Groups and Boundaries*. London: George Allen and Unwin.

Blakemore, K. and Boneham, M. (1994) *Age, Race and Ethnicity*. Buckingham: Open University Press.

Bonanno, A. and Calasanti, T. (1986) The status of rural elderly in rural southern Italy: a political economic view, *Ageing and Society*, 6(1), 13–37.

Bowling, A. and Farquar, M. (1993) The health and wellbeing of Jewish people aged 65 to 85 years living at home in the East End of London, *Ageing and Society*, 13(2), 213–44.

Brah, A. (1994) Time, place and others: discourses of race, nation, and ethnicity, *Sociology*, 28(3), 805–13.

Cantor, M. (1976) The effect of ethnicity on lifestyles of the inner-city elderly, in M. Lawton, R. Newcomer and T. Byerts (eds) *Community Planning for an Aging Society*. New York: Dowden, Hutchinson and Ross.

Chappell, N. and Marshall, V. (1992) Social integration and caregiving among seniors in Bermuda, *Ageing and Society*, 12(4), 499–514.

Checkoway, B. and Morales-Martinez, F. (1990) En La Tercera Edad: new programmes to promote the health of older people in Costa Rica, *Ageing and Society*, 10(4), 397–411.

Chetkow-Yanoov, B. (1986) Leadership among the aged: a study of engagement among third-age professionals in Israel, *Ageing and Society*, 6(1), 55–74.

Cunningham-Burley, S. (1986) Becoming a grandparent, *Ageing and Society*, 6(4), 453–70.

Davis, D. (1985) Belligerent legends: bickering and feuding among Outport octogenarians, *Ageing and Society*, 5(4), 431–48.

Dowd, J. and Bengtson, V. (1978) Aging in minority populations: an examination of the double jeopardy hypothesis, *Journal of Gerontology*, 33, 427–36.

Fennell, G., Phillipson, C. and Evers, H. (1988) *The Sociology of Old Age*. Milton Keynes: Open University Press.

Foner, N. (1973) *Status and Power in Rural Jamaica*. New York: Teachers College Press.

Foner, N. (1979) *Jamaica Farewell*. London: Routledge.

Hampson, J. (1985) Elderly people and social welfare in Zimbabwe, *Ageing and Society*, 5(1), 39–67.

Harper, S. (1987) The kinship network of the rural aged, *Ageing and Society*, 7(3), 303–27.

Harper, S. (1992) Caring for China's ageing population: the residential option – a case study of Shanghai, *Ageing and Society*, 12(2), 157–84.

Hazan, H. (1984) Religion in an old age home: symbolic adaption as a survival strategy, *Ageing and Society*, 4(2), 137–56.

Holzberg, C. (1982) Ethnicity and aging: anthropological perspectives on more than just the minority elderly, *The Gerontologist*, 33, 249–57.

Jefferys, M. (1996) Bradeley retirement village: a good thing or a bad thing?, *Generations Review*, 6(1), 5–6.

Jerrome, D. (1981) The significance of friendship for women in later life, *Ageing and Society*, 1(2), 175–97.

Jylah, M. and Jokela, J. (1990) Individual experiences as cultural – a cross-cultural study on loneliness among the elderly, *Ageing and Society*, 10(3), 295–315.

Markides, K. and Mindel, C. (1987) *Aging and Ethnicity*. London: Sage.

Matthews, S. (1983) Definitions of friendship and their consequences in old age, *Ageing and Society*, 3(2), 141–55.

Mays, N. (1983) Elderly South Asians in Britain: a survey of the literature and themes for future research, *Ageing and Society*, 3(2), 71–97.

Moller, V. (1994) Intergenerational relationships in a society in transition: a South African case study, *Ageing and Society*, 3(1), 71–97.

Nies, H., Tester, S. and Nuijens, J. (1991) Day care in the United Kingdom and the Netherlands: a comparative study, *Ageing and Society*, 11(3), 245–73.

Reid, J. (1985) 'Going up' or 'going down': the status of old people in an Australian Aboriginal society, *Ageing and Society*, 5(1), 69–95.

Rose, A. (1965) The subculture of aging: a framework in social gerontology, in A. Rose and W. Peterson (eds) *Older People in Their Social World*. Philadelphia: Davis, 3–16.

Starrett, R., Decker, J., Araujo, A. and Walters, G. (1987) The social service utilization behaviour of US Mainland Puerto Rican elderly: a causal model, *Ageing and Society*, 7(4), 445–58.

Synak, B. (1987) The elderly in Poland: an overview of selected problems and changes, *Ageing and Society*, 7(1), 19–35.

Victor, C. (1987) *Old Age in Modern Society: a Textbook of Social Gerontology*. London: Croom Helm.

Wenger, C. (1982) Ageing and rural communities: family contacts and community integration, *Ageing and Society*, 2(2), 211–29.

Wenger, C. (1985) Care in the community: changes in dependency and use of domiciliary services – a longitudinal perspective, *Ageing and Society*, 5(2), 143–59.

## 4

HANNAH ZEILIG

# The uses of literature in the study of older people

There has been a growing awareness that gerontology may have much to gain from the humanities in general. It has been increasingly appreciated that, just as Kohli (1988: 368) noted that the sociology of ageing has barely moved from its status as an applied discipline and that ageing should not be treated as a topic by itself, neither should gerontologists confine themselves to purely 'scientific' fields of research. This premise is argued cogently by Cole *et al.* (1992: 8), who state that the relevance of the humanities for ageing is that: 'we are asked to contemplate not only a proposition but the proposer . . . we hear the human voice behind what is said.' More recently the importance fictional literature in particular may have has been cited: 'What literary works can do beyond the disciplines of gerontology is to convey the experiences of ageing' (Yahnke and Eastman, 1995: 9).

Despite this increase of interest in the humanities, and literature in particular, little attempt has been made to dissect in any detail the possible ways in which such literature may be useful to gerontology. Given the multiple complexities involved in such a question (what is 'literature', what do we mean when referring to 'use' and so on), it is understandable that such issues have often not been fully addressed. In this chapter the intention is to outline some of the major theoretical debates concerning the relationship between literature and society as one way of addressing some of the questions concerning how literature may indeed be of 'use'. This is followed by a critical analysis of some recent uses of literature in gerontology; and conclusions which suggest the limitations and potential for using literature in the study of older people. The term 'literature' will be treated as applying to fiction in a broad sense; that is, written works of imagination, including novels, poems and plays.

## Some theoretical debates concerning the uses of literature in society

In order to arrive at any conclusions concerning the uses which literature might specifically have in the study of older people, it is interesting to start with some of the very broad questions which sociologists of literature have grappled with. It seems that two of the fundamental questions to which answers are sought are:

- Is it feasible to extrapolate from literature in order to gain insight into other fields of inquiry?
- If so, what can be gained from literature, what is the type of information which it can yield?

### *Goldmann and structuralism*

There has been much debate among sociologists concerning the ways in which literature can be used as a means of interpreting society, and of the interplay between literature and society (for instance, the ways in which the development of the novel is closely connected with changes in society at large). Goldmann (1967) was one of the first sociologists to explicate the relationship between literature and society in intricate detail. The somewhat obvious starting position which Goldmann takes is that thought is a part of social life, and in conjunction with this, that the human sciences cannot have such an objective character as the natural sciences. He goes on to suggest a variety of premises concerning ways in which literature is inextricably connected with society. The principal ones are:

1 The essential relationship between the life of a society and literary creation is concerned with categories which shape the empirical consciousness of a certain social group and the imaginary universe created by a writer.
2 Mental structures or (the term he prefers) 'significant categorical structures', which govern ways in which people think, are social phenomena.
3 Following logically from the last point is the idea that the relationship between the structure of a consciousness of a social group and the universe of a literary work is that of homology.

Therefore, an utterly imaginary universe, as in a fairy tale, may be strictly homologous with the experience of a particular social group or at least linked in a significant manner. Essentially what is advocated is a structuralist approach (the precise term is 'genetic structuralism').

What Goldmann has attempted to do is to prove in a quasi-scientific manner that it is perfectly feasible to extrapolate from literature as it is so intimately connected with society. The type of information which it yields would therefore presumably be reflective in a traceable sense of the structure of the society in which it was written. This is a useful perspective, and one which has informed (and continues to do so) an understanding of the ways in which literature is related to society and can legitimately be used as a means of interpreting it. Yet the fundamental implication upon which Goldmann bases the relationship – that the structure of a literary work is necessarily linked with the structure of the society in which it was written, that correspondence is never a relation of content but is in fact one of 'form' – although persuasive, is perhaps a little simplistic. It also presupposes that if the structure of a novel (for instance) is unravelled, a comprehension of the novel will follow, which may not necessarily be the case.

However, one of the most pertinent points that Goldmann makes as part of this analysis is the need to distinguish between interpretation, which is immanent to texts which are the focus of study, and explanation, which is external to texts. In other words, everything which is placed in the relationship of the text with facts which are external to it is 'explanatory' and must be judged from that standpoint. If this is accepted, it is impossible to refer to the subconscious of Orestes or the desire of Oedipus to marry his mother, as these are texts, according to Goldmann's analysis: 'the explanatory principle can reside only in the subconscious of Sophocles or Aeschylus and never in the subconscious of a literary character' (Goldmann 1967: 584). It is not, apparently, that Goldmann wishes to dismiss all psychological explanations as useless: there is an acceptance that they may account for certain aspects of a text; but these are always aspects which in the case of literature 'are not literary'. Whatever one may think contributes to literature being 'literary', Goldmann's caution about extracting one aspect of a work, especially the psychological motivations of a character, who is after all the creation of its author, and using this as the sole means of interpreting literature, is salutary.

### The didactic power of fiction

Rockwell (1977), in her analysis of the relationship between literature and society, goes one step further than Goldmann. She is interested not simply in laying bare the relationship between literature and society – how it may be a mirror of society, as Stendhal would have it – but proposes that literature is 'an essential part of the social machinery, as much an institution as any other' (Rockwell 1977: 35). Rockwell argues that the invention of narrative fiction is second only to the invention of language as a mode of transmitting the central ideas of a society to its members; as a result, literature creates a social bond on the basis of the tendency of human beings to identify with and imitate the observed action of others. In this way, the argument continues, literature is not only an interpreter of the life and norms of a society, but functionally a substitute or shadow version of them. Thus it is important in repeating and indoctrinating the norms. This is proposed as constituting the 'didactic' power of literature, which Rockwell regards as one of the implicit functions of literature. However, she admits that it is also a mirror of the wishes and dreams nurtured by a society. There is a recognition that the novel (the form of 'literature' considered in most detail by Rockwell) is an art form which necessarily selects for inspection or exploration a very small range out of the myriad of possibilities in reality, and that it cannot therefore be treated as an accurate blueprint of society at any one time. More importantly, it 'gives us a chance to perceive, if not always to understand, the values and accepted behaviour of its own time and place' (Rockwell 1977: 38).

This approach, by insisting upon firmly locating a work of literature in its own time and place, yet stressing the 'didactic' importance it may have as a channel by which the norms of that society may be handed on to its members, is another way in which 'literature' in general may be regarded as being of 'use' to other fields of inquiry. Clearly then, it is acceptable to extrapolate from literature if it is, as Rockwell would have it, an embodiment of the norms of the society which produced it. From this premise it follows that the information uncovered in the literature would be a guide to these social norms. That is, it may be used as data to look at how images and representations (for instance) of older people found in literature may reinforce or even help to create the stereotypes which we have of this section of society. A reservation which may be raised about generalizing from images found in literature, and stating that if an older person appears in a novel as a hunched up 'crone' this may be indicative of how that society perceives older people, is that there may be a danger that the individual imagination of a particular author is disregarded. After all, that author may be using a particular older person on a thoroughly symbolic level which is solely relevant within the parameters of a particular novel, poem or play.

## Cultural materialism

It is the perspective of Raymond Williams which I find most apposite when thinking about the relationship of literature to society. In *Writing in Society* (1983), he succinctly analyses the many theoretical approaches to uses of literature to illuminate society, from the Marxist view that valuable literature is that which can be judged according to its fidelity to observable social reality, to the formalists such as Bakhtin and on to his own position, which he describes as 'cultural materialism'. This involves an analysis of all forms of signification, including centrally writing, within the actual means and conditions of their production. Williams is therefore alive to the independent values of literature, but also believes that it is intrinsically associated with society. For instance, he raises the point that it was only at some time in the nineteenth century (which was late in terms of the history of literature, which might be said to span over six centuries) that the majority of the English could read and write, and states that 'It is impossible that this had no effect on what was written and what was read' (Williams 1983: 69).

Williams rails against the fact that literature is often seen as a 'specialized' area of study, believing that instead of relatively isolated forays from a specialized centre there has to be a more open and equal convergence of independent disciplines, seeking to make their evidence and their questions come together in a common inquiry. He suggests that questions which some sociological readings give of plays, poems and novels are those which ought to be central in history and sociology themselves, but which orthodox methods have failed to identify. According to Williams's analysis, as literature is evidently associated with society, it is not only feasible but also necessary to use it as a means of gaining insight into other fields of inquiry. The main tenet of belief is that literature may produce evidence which is not available elsewhere, but only if 'literature is treated as literature'. Thus, it must be read as a highly aware and articulate record of individual experience within a certain culture, and in this way it can yield important evidence. Exactly what this 'evidence' might be is never made explicit. Indeed, the greatest weakness of 'cultural materialism' as a theory is that it fails to identify in any clear way the type of information which literature may yield. On these grounds it has been criticized as failing to be an analytic theory (Harvey 1988: 24). However, the point is that Williams, in stressing the individuality of a work of literature, is unable to produce any grand theory which will adequately apply to every work. I would agree with Williams that all correlation or use of literature (be this for sociological purposes, which is what has been mainly concentrated upon, or even psychological analysis) must begin from the fact of the work. Once this is taken fully into account and the work is then related to the social context in which it was written, I think that literature may indeed, in conjunction with other disciplines, provide new insights. What these insights are will vary according to the novel, poem or play and its context.

## A critical analysis of some methods of using literature with gerontology

### King Lear and disengagement theory

When one is contemplating old age, older people and what it means to grow old, no single answer is possible, and the variety of perspectives afforded by different authors at different epochs who have tackled the subject demonstrate this. One of the main uses of literature may be to highlight both the diversity of experiences of ageing and equally possible similarities which have been expressed across time and by different cultures. Looking at one of literature's best known older characters – part historical, part mythological – was one way of considering the possibilities and limitations of using literature for gerontological purposes. My aim when thinking about *King Lear* using 'disengagement theory' was to attempt to explore how far the play might be illuminated by examination from a 'gerontological slant', and also to reappraise the theory. There are obvious problems with using a theory formulated in the late twentieth century to interpret a play written some four hundred years earlier. However, the attempt was to draw out one of the major themes of the play – Lear's decision to renounce his kingdom, and examine the extent to which this theme is explicated by gerontological theory.

*King Lear* depicts the inevitable clash between youth and age, and this forms an integral part of the tragedy of both Lear and Gloucester. It is because the prospect of an ageing father deserted by his children touches upon a raw nerve that is extant in us all that the play is so painful. However, we sympathize with both the old men and their children. It is utterly comprehensible that a father may be to his child both a loved protector and an obstructing tyrant. Conversely, to a parent the child may be a loving supporter of age, yet also a ruthless usurper and rival.

With reference to 'disengagement theory', this could be viewed as the positive desire of Regan, Goneril and Edmund for their parents to withdraw/disengage from their roles in order that they might take over. However, the theory posits that the older person also gains from such withdrawal, and that it is 'an inevitable mutual withdrawal or disengagement resulting in decreased interaction between the ageing person and others in the social system he belongs to' (Cumming and Henry 1961: 14). In giving up his kingdom, Lear's action could be interpreted as one of disengagement. From this perspective successful ageing implies: 'a reduction in activity levels and a decrease in involvement until the individual withdraws from all previous activities and becomes preoccupied with self and ultimate death' (Victor 1991: 38). At the heart of this theory, then, is the loss of the major life role. The main dilemma for Lear is that while he seems to be willingly disengaging he still wishes to be treated as a king. As a direct result of his subsequent rolelessness or 'anomie', Lear does become 'preoccupied with self', as the theory suggests. However, this has dire consequences, leading him into insanity.

This is in line with the evidence against disengagement being an adaptive process. Older people often experience a loss of roles as they age, and this is not necessarily negative. But conversely, there is little empirical evidence to support the assertion that such withdrawal is beneficial. Clearly the play revolves upon extremity, and Regan and Goneril's treatment of their father is shocking, just as Edmund's ruthlessness towards his elderly father is untenable. But to suggest that there comes a stage when it is reasonable that children take over from their fathers, who must withdraw from former roles, is not outlandish. This unhappy paradox is poignantly captured when, retorting to Regan's questioning of his need for servants, Lear bewilderedly notes, 'I gave you all', to which Regan sharply responds, 'And in good time you gave it' (Act 2, Scene 4, 246). To a certain extent Regan has reason on her side.

Thus, albeit tentatively, using *King Lear* in connection with 'disengagement theory' shows that this perspective should not be too glibly disregarded, as it can still provide some useful insights. Yet using a play in this manner is also fraught with complications. In the first instance, care must be taken when extracting themes which are apparent to the researcher, but may have minimal relevance to the work as a whole or to the audiences for whom it was intended. If a particular angle of a play is investigated, this must be acknowledged and placed in relation to the entirety of the narrative. Therefore, although the initial action of *King Lear* is ignited by Lear renouncing his kingdom, and this is therefore a feasible angle to explore, it must be recognized that it is only one aspect of the story and that in any case the story is about an extraordinary man (he was a king) who is caught up in a series of extreme situations. In this sense, the play presents an atypical example of an ageing man; although his old age may be a universally understandable phenomenon, his circumstances are not. It is not, then, that *King Lear* can be used as definitive evidence to 'prove' that disengagement theory is or is not plausible, rather that the play can provide alternative concepts with which to review the theory.

### The Death of Ivan Ilyitch

There can be serious pitfalls to the use of literature to study older people. Robert Wilson's (1995) analysis of Tolstoy's short story, *The Death of Ivan*

*Ilyitch*, highlights some of these. Wilson commences by giving a general outline of the uses which he believes literature can have, before analysing Tolstoy's short story in detail. Henry James is cited – 'the writer's first task is to make us see, to reveal life as it really is' – in support of his belief that Tolstoy excels in this; and presumably in order to bolster his use of this short story. The quote attributed to James must be treated with caution, as it is questionable to what extent any writer is able to 'reveal life as it really is'. Wilson then remarks upon Tolstoy's 'marvellous' ability to 'slip emphatically into Ilyitch's caution and conformity' (Wilson 1995: 116), despite being of a quite different temperament from Ivan Ilyitch himself. Wilson states the obvious here, for Ilyitch is a character created by Tolstoy. It was Tolstoy who built into the person of Ilyitch a certain caution and conformity, and although a novelist can feasibly be said to 'empathize' with a character, it is a rather crass truism. Lowenthal's assertion (noted by Wilson 1995: 117) that 'literature' is more real than reality itself', because we often know more about fictional characters than about people actually encountered, is not expanded further. In one sense this is true, but fictional characters are revealed to the reader, having been created and filtered through the mind of the author, and hence we know no more about them than the author wishes us to know. There is a recognition that the artist's vision should not be deformed with 'clumsy conceptual forcings' (*ibid.* 117), but the author appears to want this particular short story to represent a great deal. The opening section is concluded with a flourish: 'Ilyitch's life is all lives, his death is all deaths' (*ibid.* 117).

Although the story is well interpreted, the final section, where the author draws out 'three themes: meditations on living toward a better death' (*ibid.* 122), reveals one of the dangers of using literature. That is the tendency to want it to stand for certain 'timeless' lessons or values without much evaluation or contextualization of these. The assertion that there are three central lessons to be learnt from Ivan's story begs the question of how plausible it is to extrapolate from literature in this way. The proposition that readers in the late twentieth century can learn directly from this story in the ways set out is unsettling. Although the story had a real effect on me when I first read it, prompting thoughts about the possibility of dying with a realization that life has not been lived properly, I was simultaneously acutely aware that the death of Ivan Ilyitch was peculiar to circumstances of his time and place.

## The Picture of Dorian Gray

Kastenbaum's (1995) interpretation of Wilde's novel *The Picture of Dorian Gray* also demonstrates some of the more obvious dangers of taking a novel and using it to provide gerontological insights without proper regard for its whole context. The basic problem with using *The Picture of Dorian Gray* to explicate notions around eternal youth is that youth is used in the novel primarily as a symbol of superficiality and decadence. It is connected with Wilde's interest in aestheticism; and is not important in relation to age. Dorian's portrait reflects his moral corruption rather than how he would look if he were ageing. If literature is used effectively and in order to generate new insights, the whole story must be considered. For instance, one of the main themes in *The Picture of Dorian Gray* is the need to repress homosexuality in the late nineteenth century. Yet Kastenbaum, although attempting to put the novel 'in its own times', makes only passing mention of this, in the form of a feminist critique by a nineteenth-century woman: 'Dora Gray'. Dora Gray goes on to offer what is certainly the most original supposition of the whole book, that 'the excessive fear of ageing is not caused by homosexuality. It is more the other way around' (Kastenbaum 1995: 72).

Similarly, there is a danger with taking fictional characters out of context and treating them as though they actually existed. Hence statements such as 'Dorian's decontextualisation of youth leads to self-deception' (*ibid.* 190) are misleading; after all, Dorian Gray was *Wilde's* creation. This confusion between an author and the characters she or he has created is quite common when literature is used. It is part of what Goldmann objects to in referring to explanation being external to texts. In this case the author starts to endow the character of Dorian Gray with a life of his own.

A reading of this book highlights the care that must be taken if literature is used to enlighten gerontology. Kastenbaum is certainly inventive and imaginative, but throws together a hotch potch of literary references without any apparent criteria and then wildly formulates theories which were suggested to him from his own interpretations of the texts. For gerontologists, recourse to literature may be an important means of deepening understanding about older people, but in order fully to exploit its potential uses, limitations must also be recognized.

## Conclusions: the limitations of using literature and towards ways in which it might be used

Too often when literature is used, the impulse seems to be to make *a priori* generalizations. A novel might be able to tell us something about attitudes to older people during the time in which it was written, but the fact that it is an individual author's creation and that the response which a reader has to it is highly subjective must also be recognized. Obviously, literature exists objectively, but it exists primarily in our response to it. As David Coward (1977: 8) puts it,

> An author may speak, but we do not listen passively for we add our commentary to his monologue . . . Words have dictionary definitions but we give them a context: we give them colour and mood and meaning and their combinations acquire a significance which their first orderer may not have envisaged.

There is also an implicit assumption in some interpretations of literature that our response to it is a collective one, and the danger with this is a presupposition of the existence of final values.

Literature is above all work of imagination, it is 'fiction', which is not necessarily concerned with the facts and figures of gritty reality. On the contrary, it is often 'escapist' in nature and thus shirks what is less palatable. Burke (1973: 133) notes as part of a comment on popular 'inspirational' literature: 'It "fills a need", since there is always a need for easy consolation – and in an era of confusion like our own, the need is especially keen.' Of course, not all literature is about happy endings, neat marriages and the plot being resolved; it does not always therefore fulfil a need for easy consolation. But it is at one remove from more objective attempts to describe societal forces. Neither does fiction pertain to accurate description of individual lives, as does, for instance, biographical work. Any work of art is wholly subjective (it is the product of the imagination of a particular person within a certain social context), and this is often overlooked by critics wishing to make grandiose claims for the historical, psychological or other insights which may be gained by reading a certain novel, for instance.

If *a priori* generalizations are avoided and the subjective and fictional nature of any piece of literature is appreciated, it may begin to be useful in some of the ways which Williams (1983) advocates. Too often when literature has been used in gerontology it has been in the form of glittery anecdotes to enliven studies. In other instances, when it is the primary reference point, the analysis is intrinsically weakened when literature is used to support pre-formulated ideas. However, if literature is carefully contextualized in terms of its literary specificity (its genre and complete narrative) and historical background, then it may be an invaluable means of enriching gerontology by provoking new ways with which to consider gerontological issues.

It is impossible to outline categorical ways in which literature can lead to an understanding of issues connected with ageing because, as has been argued, this will depend upon both the work studied and its whole context. However, there are several instances where fiction has been used convincingly, albeit for very different purposes. Jill Manthorpe (1995) refers to a variety of novels in order to examine a particular institution (the private care sector) which is related to the lives of older people. Manthorpe thus gives her study a clearly delineated focus: novels written in the late twentieth century within the context of their time. There is no attempt to suggest that fiction offers the whole story and neither are extravagant claims made concerning its power to uncover profound truths about the ageing process. In this manner, Manthorpe usefully provides another means of thinking about social policy as it affects older people, through her use of fiction.

Literature has also been used in connection with psychoanalytic theory (Woodward 1991). In *Ageing and Its Discontents*, the texts are read with psychoanalytic theory in a reciprocal fashion, in order to ask what the two together can suggest about ageing. The overriding objective of the book seems to be an attempt to get at the experiences and 'anticipatory fantasies' (p. 17) of ageing, rather than simply to provide a critique of representations of ageing. In such a fashion, a dual discourse is created, whereby theory and literature work together to open up new ways of thinking about ageing. It seems to me that one of the most interesting ways of using literature with gerontology, so that it does raise questions about ageing which conventional modes of inquiry fail to do (as suggested by cultural materialism), is in conjunction with theory, as a tool with which to provoke hermeneutic inquiry. In this way, literature can function not so much as 'evidence' but as a source of data from which ideas may be extrapolated through an inductive process, with constant and meticulous regard for the fact that a highly specialized data set is being used.

## References

Burke, K. (1973) Literature as equipment for living, in E. Burns and T. Burns (eds) *The Sociology of Literature and Drama*. Harmondsworth: Penguin.

Burns, T. (1973) Introduction, in E. Burns and T. Burns (eds) *The Sociology of Literature and Drama*. Harmondsworth: Penguin.

Cole, T., Van Tassel, D. and Kastenbaum. R. (eds) (1992) *The Handbook of the Humanities and Ageing*. New York: Springer.

Coward, D. (1977) The sociology of literary response, in J. Rouff and J. Wolff (eds) *The Sociology of Literature: Theoretical Approaches*. Stafford: Wood Mitchell and Co.

Cumming, E. and Henry, W.E. (1961) *Growing Old. The Process of Disengagement*. New York: Basic Books.

Goldmann, L. (1967) Sociology of literature, status and problems of method, in M. Albrecht, J. Barnett and M. Griff (eds) *Sociology of Art and Literature. A Reader*. London: Duckworth Press.

Harvey, A.D. (1988) *Literature into History*. London: Macmillan.

Kastenbaum, R. (1995) *Dorian, Graying: Is Youth the Only Thing Worth Having?* Amityville, NY: Baywood Publishing.

Kohli, R. (1988) Ageing as a challenge for sociological theory, *Ageing and Society*, 8, 367–94.

Leavis, F.R. (1952) *The Common Pursuit*. London: Chatto and Windus.

Manthorpe, J. (1995) The private residential home in fiction, *Generations Review*, 5(1), 5–6.

Rockwell, J. (1977) A theory of literature and society, in J. Rouff and J. Wolff (eds) *The Sociology of Literature: Theoretical Approaches*. Stafford: Wood Mitchell and Co.

Victor, C. (1991) *Old Age in Modern Society*, 2nd edn. London: Chapman and Hall.

Williams, R. (1983) *Writing in Society*. London: Verso.

Wilson, R. (1995) The case of Ivan Ilyitch, *Ageing and Society*, 15, 115–24.

Woodward, K. (1991) *Aging and Its Discontents: Freud and Other Fictions*. Bloomington: Indiana University Press.

Yahnke, R. and Eastman, R. (1995) *Literature and Gerontology, a Research Guide*. New Haven, CT: Greenwood Press.

# 5

## DAVID G. TROYANSKY

# Historical research into ageing, old age and older people

History and gerontology share an interest in the passage of time. Both concern change and continuity; both raise issues of periodization. To treat them together implies some juxtaposition of lifetime and historical time. Gerontologists have demonstrated some awareness of historical change through experiences of ageing individuals and cohorts in particular circumstances, such as the Great Depression, the Second World War or post-1945 economic expansion, but they rarely explore pre-modern ageing except to find relatively 'timeless' discourses about growing old. Curiously, some historians seem to share this presentist perspective, particularly those who emphasize the unprecedented nature of the contemporary ageing of populations. Others, adhering to a more historicist appreciation of the diversity of arrangements in past societies, refuse to tell one story. Their rejection of 'master narratives' (whether of 'modernization' and degradation for elderly populations or of 'revisionism' and unmitigated progress towards retirement and the welfare state) makes it difficult to summarize 'findings' in the historical literature. Nevertheless, an awareness of that literature may immunize social gerontologists against incorporating overly simple ideas about change and continuity into their search for new theoretical understandings in their discipline.

This chapter begins with a consideration of the literature that organizes the recent history of ageing and old age around the concerns of historical demography. It distinguishes between ageing and old age as objects of historical investigation and then moves to works, often on the more distant past, that privilege either cultural representations of old age or social historical experiences of older people. It concludes with the recent scholarly trend of investigating history and memory.

## Historical demography and ageing

Peter Laslett (1989) provides a demographic framework for understanding the implications of the history of ageing. He describes the ageing of populations as an essential transformation in contemporary history and recommends giving it as important a place as historians have commonly given the well-known demographic transitions of falling mortality and fertility. But while those transitions have origins going back to the eighteenth century, demographic ageing has a shorter history, and Laslett emphasizes the dramatic shift occurring after 1950, which saw the generalization of an entirely new stage of the life-course. The 'third age' consists of the young old, who retire early enough and in sufficiently good health to enjoy an unprecedented period of cultivation, creativity and leisure. The emergence of Laslett's third age coincided with a period of economic growth, expanding educational and leisure opportunities, and state intervention in the form of social security.

Some forms of the third age have existed in the past for relatively small numbers of people, whose experiences have been featured in histories of old age. The democratization of that experience in 'age-transformed' populations is key to Laslett's periodization, but even in the contemporary period, demographic ageing alone does not explain the historical experience of older people. Specialists in the period have emphasized the role of the state, not only as responding to social needs, but also in creating new demands. They have considered retirement as a way of managing the workforce, explored the development of a medical system that focuses on an older population and even begun to investigate the history of gerontology as a discipline.

Laslett takes an optimistic view of the opportunities for age-transformed populations and individuals in the third age. His optimism contrasts with the alarmist tone of much demographic study in the twentieth century. The very invention of the idea of demographic ageing brought with it a prejudice against advanced age. Patrice Bourdelais (1993) demonstrates the fears of early twentieth-century French demographers, who discovered the causal connection between falling fertility and population ageing. Older people became living symbols of empty cradles. Women might then be seen by male demographers as both the cause and, in recognition of the increasing female majority at the greatest ages, an effect of this process. Bourdelais also warns against the seemingly intuitive connection between demographic ageing and ideas of old age. By seeking to find equivalent chronological ages for the onset of old age – a sixty-year-old today is not the equivalent of a sixty-year-old two centuries ago – he identifies a moving threshold that removes some of the drama in the changing composition of the population. He joins Laslett in avoiding the alarm over ageing, but he is sceptical of the reliance on historical demography in the absence of social, political and cultural history.

## Family and household

Laslett came to the study of ageing through his work with the Cambridge Group for the History of Population and Social Structure. Their concern for the history of household formation and the family set the agenda for much modern social history, including the history of ageing, and some scholars have generalized from English historical experience to a north-western European model of the family. But generalizations about the nuclear family, which would have encouraged independence (or neglect) of older people and allegedly set north-western Europeans apart from others in the world, have been challenged by scholars discovering more complex forms. A collaborative work edited by Laslett and anthropologist–historian David Kertzer reveals considerable co-residence of adult generations in ageing households in Europe and North America (Kertzer and Laslett 1995). It transcends the old battle between proponents of nuclear and stem family models but still focuses on family and household in proposing a 'nuclear reincorporation household system' by which older persons either move in with children or are joined by them. In other words, families in early modern and modern Western societies have demonstrated great flexibility, and even in England into the twentieth century it was more common for older people to co-reside with children than to live alone or with non-relatives (Wall 1995).

If 'nuclear reincorporation' is to become the dominant interpretive model for ageing households and family history, it will have to incorporate both economic and cultural determinants of co-residence or independence (Andorka 1995; Plakans and Wetherell 1995). Sharecropping in central Italy encouraged multiple family households, so widowhood did not mean isolation as it would have in the south, where nuclear households meant greater pressure to remarry. Even after proletarianization had transformed the central Italian economy, however, widows still decided to live with married sons, a pattern that contrasts with an English one of residing with married daughters (Kertzer and Karweit 1995). Different frontier settings saw a range of adaptations in the United States (Gutmann 1995; D.S. Smith 1995), where increasing national rates of home ownership by age (Haines and Goodman 1995), the accumulation of savings and the purchase of insurance indicate strategies for achieving old age security (Ransom and Sutch 1995).

## From the history of ageing to the history of old age

A focus on local settings and particular populations moves the literature farther from the master narratives. Indeed, to understand cultural continuity and change we must extend the analysis back before the 'secular shift'. For all the novelty in an age-transformed world, neither old age nor its history was invented yesterday. The first historians of old age, writing in the 1970s and 1980s, were obviously stimulated by the demographic changes in the contemporary world, but they found social and cultural changes in earlier historical settings. They avoided the tendency to present the pre-transition past as almost undifferentiated.

### Made in the USA

Some of the first efforts in the field were undertaken by American historians, who tended to focus on what they took to be changes associated with 'modernization'. Carole Haber and Brian Gratton's (1994) survey of the American historiography conveniently divides the research into three phases. The first examined the cultural experience of modernization. The second concerned the socio-economic status of the aged in the era of industrialization. The third explored the role of the state.

In their first phase, American historians described changing attitudes. They wrote a history of decline from some form of gerontocracy to some form of ageism, but they disagreed over periodization. David Hackett Fischer (1978) described a 'deep change' between the 1770s and 1820s, whereby political power and cultural authority devolved upon the young or middle-aged. Fischer examined patterns of office-holding, the arrangement of individuals in family portraits and a range of other indicators. For Andrew Achenbaum (1978), the big change came after the Civil War, when, he claimed, old age was seen as obsolescence. But already other scholars were demonstrating that in the earlier period authority and respect depended upon control of property (Greven 1970; Demos 1986). So even in the first phase of research, historians were trying to balance social and cultural sources. Haber (1983) described the world of medicine and the medicalization of social institutions; Thomas Cole (1992) examined the interplay of religious and social thought. Both examined how changes long associated with modernization were mediated in particular cultural settings. How did medicine define old age? How did religious thinkers shift their ideas to keep up with the demands of middle-class urban life? In this historical literature, representations, discourses and attitudes (terms applied with varying degrees of specificity and difference) often had lives of their own.

The second phase saw a discussion of socio-economic conditions. The Cambridge approach to family history has its equivalent in American work describing the family and household in the era of industrialization. Some of this literature found few changes in the social experience of ageing family members. Some found the development of more complex household structures that often seemed to benefit the aged (Hareven 1982; Ruggles 1987). A debate raged among economic historians over labour-force participation (Gratton 1986). The issue mattered in addressing whether older workers were marginalized as victims of social change and ageism or whether they were finding ways of achieving retirement. But it was not an either/or proposition. In the former case, the aged were the objects of historical transformations. In the latter, they were the subjects, actors themselves.

The third phase involved a rethinking of the state as an independent actor. Rather than seeing social security as a response to a real need, it was a stimulus to other changes and encouraged the development of the third age. Historians of the American welfare state contrasted that institution with the European varieties, which emerged earlier and provided more extensive coverage. They explored the place of older people among the needy in general, the importance of management of the workforce and the expectations of different class and ethnic groups. But the most important characteristic of the third phase of research was the emphasis on a political context (Graebner 1980; Quadagno 1988; Skocpol 1992). Haber and Gratton's (1994) three-phase approach to the historical literature makes it seem that the political superseded the social, which had superseded the cultural – a reversal of the tendency in other areas of historical scholarship – but important contributions continue to be made in all such areas, including letter-writing by ageing women in the early republic (Premo 1990) and relations between older women and younger men (Banner 1992).

### A European difference

The initial American assumption that the history of old age was all about decline was not shared in the European literature, where opinions varied from seeing the lot of older persons as continuously awful to recognizing some improvement in the contemporary era. Simone de Beauvoir (1972) (not a historian but influential all the same) told a tale of never-ending woe. Peter Stearns (1976) wrote more responsibly about traditional ageism in France, and edited a collection of articles on pre-industrial societies that expressed none of the nostalgia of the first American histories (Stearns 1982). Others, recognizing a tradition of gerontophobia in European culture, wrote about the construction of a modern respect for old age in France (Gutton 1988; Bois 1989; Troyansky 1989) and Germany (Borscheid 1987) in the eighteenth century.

The important point was that the deference some took to be natural was culturally constructed. The danger, identified most recently by Pat Thane (1995), was that just as gerontologists might express optimistic or pessimistic views as a way of addressing public opinion or pleading for greater funding in an emergency, so historians sometimes opted for fairly simple narratives. Thane points out that the stories historians have told conform to standard conventions, whose choice might express hopes and fears of historians concerning old age that differed little from those of other writers in the past. But if we go too far with her critique, we risk ignoring the predominance of certain views in particular historical settings. We need not opt for some vague spirit of the times or ideas that are simply 'out there'. In examining the cultural historical literature, we must try to keep track of where our sources come from, whose attitudes they express, and where alternative views might be found.

### Culture

Georges Minois's (1989) history of old age from the ancient world to the sixteenth century is emblematic of early attempts at surveying the landscape, for it tends to slide back and forth between cultural and social approaches. Minois plays with ideas of the relative security of older people based upon their percentage of the total population and with representations of elders in different social, cultural and political contexts. He offers little, however, on household structure, family types or control of property. His strength lies in his treatment of a great variety of topics under the rubric of old age: population, religion, art, death, medicine, retirement, the state, etc. He tries to avoid anachronism by asking how the very idea of old age was constituted in the past rather than applying twentieth-century definitions. His survey of testimony about individual lives, prescriptive literature on how one ought to age and graphic representations of classic tropes of youth and age reveals ambiguities from the ancient past to the Renaissance.

Minois is not a specialist in the ancient world. His version of antiquity serves to prepare the way for the rebirth of classical knowledge in the Renaissance and after. His classical past sets up polar opposites of respect and disdain for old age. The ambiguity was there from the start, and he traces it through time. Among the Hebrews, elders are honourable and close to the sacred, but that position declines, particularly under Hellenistic influence. Christianity partook of this emphasis on youth – this was a way of distinguishing itself from Judaism and also a way of representing the youthful soul versus the aged body – but even there we can find the theme of the good, aged (and young) widow (Mirrer 1992; Bremmer and Bosch 1995). These are literary discourses, and the subject position may vary (ageing individuals writing about themselves or, more commonly, younger people writing about their elders), but we are given ingredients that will be combined in different ways. Thus, Plato's Cephalus is the idealized, virtuous old man, and Aristotle's old age is a time of foolishness. Old age may be an occasion for tragedy and the butt of comedy, but for the Greek world we are dealing almost exclusively with literary representations, not with social realities (Falkner and de Luce 1992). None the less, entry into old age for women seems to have been associated with menopause, while the marker for men was more social or generational.

Rome provides similar cultural ambiguities, but developments in legal and political history resulted in the creation of more usable sources. It also produced the most famous apologia for old age, Cicero's *De Senectute*, whose history in the early modern period has drawn some attention. But that is a description of an elite public man. Poetic treatment of ageing and lascivious women in Horace or Juvenal is something altogether different. Tim Parkin (1995), a specialist in the ancient world, has warned against over-interpretation from limited data, but recognizes that sources for social reality exist. For him, the status of the aged depended upon individual abilities, and the ambiguities are similar to those in the modern era.

Minois's medieval world brings into play several themes that will recur. One is the Christian emphasis on youth, but often youth and age represented metaphysical categories, and philosophers described an idealized course of life. Nevertheless, the Church sometimes provided a privileged space for older people to exercise their holiness and their talents for organization. Minois also shows how older persons were relatively secure from the plague, thus creating social situations where the aged might dominate. Shulamith Shahar (1995) argues that medical discourses on ageing were among the most tolerant, as decline is seen as no fault of the individual. On the other hand, she sees a cruelty in religious texts. But even there ageing provided an opportunity for concentration on the soul and transcendence.

Medieval representations of the ages of life had a long-lasting cultural impact (Sheehan 1990). Throughout the Western world, images of the life course as a ladder presented a model at several levels of culture (Burrow 1986; Sears 1986). Stereotypes of an eighty- or one-hundred-year life may have corresponded poorly to real experience, but the representation of forty or fifty years of ascent and forty or fifty years of decline provided a powerful metaphorical structure that transcended national differences. Thus, *Die Lebenstreppe* or *les degrés des âges* provided a model into the twentieth century (*Die Lebenstreppe* 1983). Other stereotypes continued to appear, juxtaposing youth and age and enforcing social and sexual norms (Wildt and Ham 1993).

Paralleling the work of Minois in France, but dispensing with the survey of the ancient and medieval eras, is Peter Borscheid's (1987) work on early modern Germany. While he provides more than Minois on family and household structure, his categories are very much the literary/moral ones. Indeed, he briefly compares Catholic and Protestant views, with a Reformed German culture encouraging the emergence of a kind of patriarchy in which the father is a stand-in for God. In Borscheid's account, patriarchy is encouraged even more in the rebuilding of central European society after the Thirty Years' War. But this time the key institution cuts across confessional differences, as his story of the civilization process is one of a powerful nation state. Parental authority parallels absolutist authority.

Borscheid's eighteenth century still features a large role for religion in the Pietist desire to reform the world. However, most work on that period emphasizes secularization and the Enlightenment, when representations of old age demonstrated a shift from ridicule to respect. This does not mean that behaviour changed in any particular way but it does mark a shift in image. It is probably the case that such cultural shifts had an impact on 'ordinary' people's thoughts and actions. This chronology fits nicely with that of the history of childhood and the family. It confirms the idea of a 'creation' of man, society and modern politics. Institutions of the French Revolutionary period suggest a new social view that some see as anticipating the welfare state.

The constitution of old age as both a stage in the life course and a social problem has occupied historians working on the period since the eighteenth century. Investigations of high culture reveal an unprecedented concern for old age in the second half of the eighteenth century, a reaction against comic ridicule of older persons and the articulation of myths of founding fathers or elders. It is as if an awareness of historical change encouraged a new appreciation of elders, whether founding fathers in the USA or older people in French Revolutionary festivals. A similar constellation of circumstances emerges a bit later in Australia, where historians have described youth and age in the creation of national self-images and the development of 'ageism' in a frontier, colonial society. By the 1890s, gold rush immigrants in their sixties made pioneer days seem old rather than youthful (Davison 1995). Alternatively, one might push Australian ageism back to the 'traditional' world of the early nineteenth century (Karskens 1995).

Some cultural historians recommend age as one useful category among many. The study of nineteenth-century suicide by age raises questions of past medical and legal ideas of rationality (Cooke 1995). A treatment of nineteenth- and twentieth-century feminism emphasizes intergenerational debate (Caine 1995). In these and other recent treatments, we find an interest in the way fields of thought and knowledge are defined. Gerontology itself, as a multidisciplinary enterprise of physicians, biologists, social scientists, foundations, universities and government agencies, always involved crossing boundaries (Achenbaum 1995). But it has generally leaned more to the social sciences than the humanities.

## Society

In surveying historical scholarship on ageing and the aged, Paul Johnson (1995) contends that cultural history has operated in a relativistic paradigm. In the social history that he describes as more positivistic he identifies three major themes: participation, well-being and status, all classic social historical categories weighted towards issues of employment, property ownership and transmission of household authority. These issues have been crucial in the development of a history of old age in England (Pelling and Smith 1991), which has explored how early modern collectivities dealt with issues of responsibility for ageing residents (R.M. Smith 1995; *Ageing and Society* 1984), how families shared out children in ageing households (Pelling 1991) and how periods of bereavement lengthened in the eighteenth century (Wright 1991). For Johnson, functional capacity and control of property were essential to the maintenance of authority in virtually all historical contexts, but differences, particularly in the modern era, have often resulted from the impact of institutions. In Germany, Josef Ehmer's social history (1990) is all about social policy, demands by organized labour, working-class households and the welfare state. Recent French social history has focused on the emergence of modern retirement, which became almost everyone's way of managing old age, as the ideas of political parties, labour unions and interest groups converged at the turn of the century (Pollet 1990). Often civil servants led private-sector workers in discovering retirement (Dumons 1990). The social historical literature has been influenced by sociologists like Martin Kohli (1986) and Anne-Marie Guillemard, who have described retirement as a way of managing old age in a world of work. But recent evidence of a greater separation between retirement and old age has thrown this literature into some disarray (Guillemard *et al.* 1995). The institutionalization of old age as retirement has been succeeded by a rapid deinstitutionalization.

None the less, questions about career, retirement and public institutions need to be placed in a long-term historical context. Scholars in Europe and the United States have found complex and gradual patterns of 'stepping down' (Held 1982; Kertzer and Schaie 1989). Even in the absence of national social security schemes, aged English paupers in the early nineteenth century fashioned identities to present in writing to local authorities (Sokoll 1993).

Fashioning an identity in old age has been encouraged by all sorts of institutions, particularly the state. The familiar part of the story is that of how the state left its mark on society; less familiar is the story of how people used the state. Setters of bureaucratic rules determined to a large extent how people approached the state with their life histories and demands for pensions. But the state was not so completely in control of how people making demands reconstructed their lives. It created an opportunity for relatively privileged individuals to create a sense of their own lives as coherent and meaningful.

The development of state institutions and ideas of career are important in the secularization of the life review or life history.

The history of formal pensions is only beginning to be written. Guy Thuillier (1994) has been exploring the bureaucratic angle on French pensions in the nineteenth century and has distinguished between recompense and right, but has still written policy history while hinting tantalizingly at something more. Christoph Conrad (1994), who has surveyed the German situation and focused particularly on the Rhineland and the Bismarck pensions, goes farther. Rather than writing exclusively from the point of view of the bureaucracy, he has explored pensions from the perspective of the working-class household. He rejects the idea that social policies were designed simply to meet unprecedented needs. He shows how the Bismarck pensions stimulated discussion and how working-class elders effectively cobbled together an existence. However, political actors became convinced of real needs, and they slowly brought into being the institutions of the welfare state. Old age became defined as one of many social problems in the Weimar period, when pensioners became new client groups of the state and old people moved to the centre of the health care system. Conrad (1995a) has argued that income packaging from private and public sources gives the lie to any simple private-to-public history of the welfare state. He has provided evidence of an ageing of the population receiving hospital treatment (Conrad 1995b), thus going beyond the literature's usual emphasis on medical ideas (Kondratowitz 1991; Katz 1995).

Conrad's work is indicative of research recasting the debate on the origins of the welfare state and combining elements of social and cultural history (Pedersen 1993). For labour leaders, retirement was often a diversion (Pollet 1990); for workers in the nineteenth century, barely a possibility (Melchers 1995). For businessmen, workers' pensions permitted a new kind of management of the workforce (Ransom *et al.* 1993). Detailed study of particular retiring groups in the contemporary period has indicated a process of acculturation as workers learn to anticipate and enjoy retirement (Cribier 1995). Work beginning on the early twentieth-century Parisian transit industry has provided clues about life experiences (Feller 1994). Workers writing to bureaucrats describe the intersection between careers, family histories, and such events as the First World War and the Great Depression. They reveal career histories, migration patterns and the operation of family networks in negotiating the rapidly changing Parisian world. Letters recounting lives and claiming entitlements reveal cultural meanings even in the paper generated by a developing modern bureaucracy (Troyansky 1995). Demands for retirement prompt memories of careers and personal histories.

## History and memory

The theme of memory brings us back to the relationship between gerontology and history. At first we might think that while gerontology respects memory, history seeks to correct it (Kaminsky 1984). Yet historians have been paying closer attention to the function of memory and coming to appreciate the subjective element not only in reminiscence but also in the writing of history. If historians, influenced by various forms of cultural studies, have begun to deny any privileged perspective on events, they see the meaning of those events in multiple witnesses' observations and understandings. The theme of memory has inspired intellectual and cultural historians (Hutton 1993), a new scholarly journal, *History and Memory*, is devoted to the theme, and oral history has played an essential role in the writing of social history.

Despite the fact that oral history interviews have often, for obvious reasons, been held with elderly informants, they have rarely been concerned with the informants' own ageing or even with memories of others as older persons. In a popular vein, Ronald Blythe (1979) in England and Studs Terkel (1995) in the United States have made the transition from asking older informants about a world that is lost to asking them about themselves. In a more scholarly vein, researchers have discovered reappropriations of older religious discourses (Williams 1990) and sometimes surprisingly positive subjective images of ageing (Thompson *et al.* 1990; Cribier 1995). For the contemporary history of old age, oral histories provide access to family decisions, testimony about values, ideas of who benefits from co-residence and the nature of intergenerational connections between households (Hareven and Uhlenberg 1995). Oral history sheds light on pre-revolutionary Russia and China, on fascism and the Holocaust, on repetition of 'family scripts' from generation to generation and on influences running forwards and backwards between generations (Bertaux and Thompson 1993). Memory links public and private history, and memories of public events and private life reveal important aspects of the experience of ageing. Informants' testimony falls somewhere between the images and discourses of the cultural historians and the anonymous populations of the social historians and demographers. Gerontologists who have viewed writing as a part of the life review have created sources equivalent to those of the historian. By encouraging elderly people to recount their lives and the history they have lived (see, for example, Jeffery's account in this volume), gerontologists are preserving voices other than those of the social scientific experts, the kinds of voices historians of old age would love to hear from the past (Kamler and Feldman 1995).

## Acknowledgement

This chapter draws on a previously published article by David G. Troyansky published in 1996 by Cambridge University Press, called Progress report: the history of old age in the western world, in *Ageing and Society*, 16: 233–43.

## References

Achenbaum, W.A. (1978) *Old Age in the New Land*. Baltimore: Johns Hopkins University Press.
Achenbaum, W.A. (1995) *Crossing Frontiers: Gerontology Emerges as a Science*. Cambridge: Cambridge University Press.

*Ageing and Society* (1984) Special issue: History and Ageing, 4.

Andorka, R. (1995) Household systems and the lives of the old in eighteenth- and nine-teenth-century Hungary, in D.I. Kertzer and P. Laslett (eds) *Aging in the Past: Demography, Society, and Old Age*. Berkeley: University of California Press, 129–55.

Banner, L.W. (1992) *In Full Flower: Aging Women, Power, and Sexuality, a History*. New York: Knopf.

Beauvoir, S. de (1972) *Old Age*. London: Deutsch.

Bertaux, D. and Thompson, P. (1993) *Between Generations: Family Models, Myths, and Memories. International Yearbook of Oral History and Life Stories, Vol. 2*. Oxford: Oxford University Press.

Blythe, R. (1979) *The View in Winter: Reflections on Old Age*. New York: Harcourt Brace Jovanovich.

Bois, J.-P. (1989) *Les vieux de Montaigne aux premières retraites*. Paris: Fayard.

Borscheid, P. (1987) *Geschichte des Alters 16.–18. Jahrhundert*. Münster: Coppenrath.

Bourdelais, P. (1993) *Le nouvel âge de la vieillesse: Histoire du vieillissement de la population*. Paris: Odile Jacob.

Bremmer, J. and Bosch, L. van den (1995) *Between Poverty and the Pyre: Moments in the History of Widowhood*. London: Routledge.

Burrow, J.A. (1986) *The Ages of Man: a Study in Medieval Writing and Thought*. Oxford: Clarendon Press.

Caine, B. (1995) Generational conflict and the question of ageing in nineteenth and twentieth century feminism, *Australian Cultural History*, 14, 92–108.

Cole, T.R. (1992) *The Journey of Life: a Cultural History of Aging in America*. Cambridge: Cambridge University Press.

Cole, T.R., Van Tassel, D.D. and Kastenbaum, R. (eds) (1992) *Handbook of the Humanities and Aging*. New York: Springer.

Conrad, C. (1994) *Vom Greis zum Rentner: Der Strukturwandel des Alters in Deutschland zwischen 1830 und 1930*. Göttingen: Vandenhoeck & Ruprecht.

Conrad, C. (1995a) *Income Packaging in Historical Perspective: Public and Private Support for the Elderly in Germany, 1890s–1950s*. Center for European Studies Working Paper Series. Cambridge, MA: Harvard University.

Conrad, C. (1995b) Old age and the health system in the nineteenth and twentieth centuries. Paper delivered to 18th International Congress of Historical Sciences.

Conrad, C. and Kondratowitz, H.-J. von (eds) (1993) *Zur Kulturgeschichte des Alterns/Toward a Cultural History of Aging*. Berlin: Deutsches Zentrum für Altersfragen e.V.

Cooke, S. (1995) 'Terminal old age': ageing and suicide in Victoria, 1841–1921, *Australian Cultural History*, 14, 76–91.

Cribier, F. (1995) Passage à la retraite et parcours de vie: L'exemple de deux cohortes de nouveaux retraités parisiens de 1972 et 1984, in A.-M. Guillemard *et al.* (eds) *Entre travail, retraite et vieillesse: Le grand écart*. Paris: L'Harmattan, 177–96.

Davison, G. (1995) 'Our youth is spent and our backs are bent': the origins of Australian Ageism, *Australian Cultural History*, 14, 40–62.

Demos, J.P. (1986) *Past, Present, and Personal: the Family and the Life Course in American History*. New York and Oxford: Oxford University Press.

Dumons, B. (1990) *Les retraites sous la Troisième République: Lyon et sa région (1880–1914). Population, modes de vie et comportements*. Lyon: Université de Lyon 2.

Ehmer, J. (1990) *Sozialgeschichte des Alters*. Frankfurt: Suhrkamp.

Falkner, T.M. and de Luce, J. (1992) A view from antiquity: Greece, Rome, and elders, in T.R. Cole *et al.* (eds) *Handbook of the Humanities and Aging*. New York: Springer, 3–39.

Feller, E. (1994) *Agents et retraités des transports parisiens: Trajectoires individuelles et change-ment social dans l'entre-deux-guerres*. Mémoires et Documents. Paris: Mission Archives de la RATP.

Fischer, D.H. (1978) *Growing Old in America*. New York and Oxford: Oxford University Press.

Graebner, W. (1980) *A History of Retirement: the Meaning and Function of an American Institution, 1885–1975*. New Haven, CT: Yale University Press.

Gratton, B. (1986) *Urban Elders: Family, Work, and Welfare among Boston's Aged, 1890–1950*. Philadelphia: Temple University Press.

Greven, P. (1970) *Four Generations: Population, Land, and Family in Colonial Andover, Massachusetts*. Ithaca, NY, and London: Cornell University Press.

Guillemard, A.-M., Légaré, J. and Ansart, P. (eds) (1995) *Entre travail, retraite et vieillesse: Le grand écart*. Paris: L'Harmattan.

Gutmann, M.P. (1995) Older lives on the frontier: the residential patterns of the older population of Texas, 1850–1910, in D.I. Kertzer and P. Laslett (eds) *Aging in the Past: Demography, Society, and Old Age*. Berkeley: University of California Press, 175–202.

Gutton, J.-P. (1988) *Naissance du vieillard: Essai sur l'histoire des rapports entre les vieillards et la société en France*. Paris: Aubier.

Haber, C. (1983) *Beyond Sixty-five: the Dilemma of Old Age in America's Past*. Cambridge: Cambridge University Press.

Haber, C. and Gratton, B. (1994) *Old Age and the Search for Security: an American Social History*. Bloomington and Indianapolis: Indiana University Press.

Haines, M.R. and Goodman, A.C. (1995) A home of one's own: aging and home ownership in the United States in the late nineteenth and early twentieth century, in D.I. Kertzer and P. Laslett (eds) *Aging in the Past*. Berkeley: University of California Press, 203–26.

Hareven, T. (1982) *Family Time and Industrial Time: the Relationship between Family and Work in a New England Industrial Community*. Cambridge: Cambridge University Press.

Hareven, T.K. and Uhlenberg, P. (1995) Transition to widowhood and family support systems in the twentieth century, Northeastern United States, in D.I. Kertzer and P. Laslett (eds) *Aging in the Past*. Berkeley: University of California Press, 273–99.

Held, T. (1982) Rural retirement arrangements in seventeenth to nineteenth-century Austria: a cross-community analysis, *Journal of Family History*, 7, 227–54.

Hutton, P. (1993) *History as an Art of Memory*. Hanover, NH: University Press of New England.

Johnson, P. (1995) Report: old age and aging, *Proceedings of the 18th International Congress of Historical Sciences*, 263–76.

Kaminsky, M. (1984) *The Uses of Reminiscence*. New York: Haworth Press.

Kamler, B. and Feldman, S. (1995) Mirror, mirror on the wall: reflections on ageing, *Australian Cultural History*, 14, 1–22.

Karskens, G. (1995) Declining life: on the rocks in early Sydney, *Australian Cultural History*, 14, 63–75.

Katz, S. (1995) Disciplinary texts: rhetoric and the science of old age in the late nineteenth and early twentieth centuries, *Australian Cultural History*, 14, 109–26.

Kertzer, D.I. and Karweit, N. (1995) The impact of widowhood in nineteenth-century Italy, in D.I. Kertzer and P. Laslett (eds) *Aging in the Past*. Berkeley: University of California Press, 229–48.

Kertzer, D.I. and Laslett, P. (eds) (1995) *Aging in the Past: Demography, Society, and Old Age*. Berkeley: University of California Press.

Kertzer, D.I. and Schaie, W.K. (1989) *Age Structuring in Comparative Perspective*. Hillsdale, NJ: Lawrence Erlbaum Associates.

Kohli, M. (1986) The world we forgot: a historical review of the life course, in V.W. Marshall (ed.) *Later Life: the Social Psychology of Aging*. Beverly Hills, CA: Sage Publications, 271–303.

Kondratowitz, H.-J. von (1991) The medicalization of old age: continuity and change in Germany from the late eighteenth to the early twentieth century, in M. Pelling and R.M. Smith (eds) *Life, Death, and the Elderly*. London: Routledge, 134–64.

Laslett, P. (1989) *A Fresh Map of Life: the Emergence of the Third Age*. London: Weidenfeld and Nicolson.

*Die Lebenstreppe* (1983) *Bilder der menschlichen Lebensalter*. Cologne: Rheinland-Verlag.

Melchers, R. (1995) Début de l'ère industrielle et rapports intergénérationnels dans le milieu de travail, in A.-M. Guillemard *et al.* (eds) *Entre travail, retraite et vieillesse*. Paris: L'Harmattan, 105–20.

Minois, G. (1989) *History of Old Age: from Antiquity to the Renaissance*. Cambridge: Polity Press.

Mirrer, L. (1992) *Upon My Husband's Death: Widows in the Literature and Histories of Medieval Europe*. Ann Arbor: University of Michigan Press.

Parkin, T.G. (1995) Ageing in antiquity: participation, well-being, and status. Paper delivered to 18th International Congress of Historical Sciences.

Pedersen, S. (1993) *Family, Dependence, and the Origins of the Welfare State: Britain and France, 1914–1945*. Cambridge: Cambridge University Press.

Pelling, M. (1991) Old age, poverty, and disability in early modern Norwich: work, remarriage, and other expedients, in M. Pelling and R.M. Smith (eds) *Life, Death, and the Elderly*. London: Routledge, 74–101.

Pelling, M. and Smith, R.M. (eds) (1991) *Life, Death, and the Elderly: Historical Perspectives*. London: Routledge.

Plakans, A. and Wetherell, C. (1995) Migration in the later years of life in traditional Europe, in D.I. Kertzer and P. Laslett (eds) *Aging in the Past*. Berkeley: University of California Press, 156–74.

Pollet, G. (1990) *Les retraites en France, 1880–1914: la naissance d'une politique sociale*. Lyon: Université de Lyon 2.

Premo, T.L. (1990) *Winter Friends: Women Growing Old in the New Republic, 1785–1835*. Urbana: University of Illinois Press.

Quadagno, J. (1988) *The Transformation of Old Age Security: Class and Politics in the American Welfare State*. Chicago: University of Chicago Press.

Ransom, R.L. and Sutch, R. (1995) The impact of aging on the employment of men in American working-class communities at the end of the nineteenth century, in D.I. Kertzer and P. Laslett (eds) *Aging in the Past*. Berkeley: University of California Press, 303–27.

Ransom, R., Sutch, R. and Williamson, S.H. (1993) Inventing pensions: the origins of the company-provided pension in the United States, 1900–1940, in A. Achenbaum and W.K. Schaie (eds) *Societal Impact on Aging: Historical Perspectives*. New York: Springer, 1–38.

Ruggles, S. (1987) *Prolonged Connections: the Rise of the Extended Family in Nineteenth-century England and America*. Madison: University of Wisconsin Press.

Sears, E. (1986) *The Ages of Man: Medieval Interpretations of the Life Cycle*. Princeton, NJ: Princeton University Press.

Shahar, S. (1995) The status of the elderly in the high and late Middle Ages. Paper delivered to 18th International Congress of Historical Sciences.

Sheehan, M.M. (1990) *Aging and the Aged in Medieval Europe*. Toronto: Pontifical Institute of Mediaeval Studies.

Skocpol, T. (1992) *Protecting Soldiers and Mothers: the Political Origins of Social Policy in the United States*. Cambridge, MA: Harvard University Press.

Smith, D.S. (1995) The demography of widowhood in preindustrial New Hampshire, in D.I. Kertzer and P. Laslett (eds) *Aging in the Past*. Berkeley: University of California Press, 249–72.

Smith, R.M. (1995) Ageing and well-being in early modern England. Paper delivered to 18th International Congress of Historical Sciences.

Sokoll, T. (1993) Armut im Alter im Spiegel englischer Armenbriefe des ausgehenden 18. und frühen 19. Jahrhunderts, in C. Conrad and H.-J. von Kondratowitz (eds) *Zur Kulturgeschichte des Alterns*. Berlin: Deutsches Zentrum für Altersfragen e.V., 39–76.

Stearns, P.N. (1976) *Old Age in European Society: the Case of France*. New York: Holmes and Meier.

Stearns, P.N. (1982) *Old Age in Preindustrial Society*. New York: Holmes and Meier.

Terkel, S. (1995) *Coming of Age: the Story of Our Century by Those Who've Lived it*. New York: New Press.

Thane, P. (1995) The cultural history of old age, *Australian Cultural History*, 14, 23–39.

Thompson, P., Itzin, C. and Abendstern, M. (1990) *I Don't Feel Old: the Experience of Later Life*. Oxford: Oxford University Press.

Thuillier, G. (1994) *Les pensions de retraite des fonctionnaires au XIXe siècle*. Paris: Comité d'Histoire de la Sécurité Sociale.

Troyansky, D.G. (1989) *Old Age in the Old Regime: Image and Experience in Eighteenth-century France*. Ithaca, NY, and London: Cornell University Press.

Troyansky, D.G. (1995) Retraite, vieillesse et contrat social: l'exemple des juges de la Haute-Vienne sous la Restauration, in A.-M. Guillemard *et al.* (eds) *Entre travail, retraite et vieillesse*. Paris: L'Harmattan, 85–101.

Wall, R. (1995) Elderly persons and members of their households in England and Wales from preindustrial times to the present, in D.I. Kertzer and P. Laslett (eds) *Aging in the Past*. Berkeley: University of California Press, 81–106.

Wildt, A. de and Ham, W. van der (1993) *Tijd van Leven: Ouder worden in Nederland vroeger en nu*. Amsterdam: Amsterdams Historisch Museum.

Williams, R. (1990) *A Protestant Legacy: Attitudes to Death and Illness among Older Aberdonians*. Oxford: Clarendon Press.

Wright, S.J. (1991) The elderly and the bereaved in eighteenth-century Ludlow, in M. Pelling and R.M. Smith (eds) *Life, Death, and the Elderly*. London: Routledge, 102–33.

# 6 EILEEN FAIRHURST

## Recalling life: analytical issues in the use of 'memories'

The life history method is gaining increasing currency in gerontological research. Its claimed strength is of offering a purchase on the ways in which personal biography and social history have implications for everyday features of later life. The past is seen to have a significance for understanding the present lives of older people. Moreover, plundering the past is endowed with a therapeutic purpose in reminiscence therapy. Life history narratives rest upon recall of the past and it is the elaboration and explication of that matter that is the concern of this chapter. Proponents of the life history method identify its distinctiveness in terms of its concerns with concepts such as the self and identity. The very stuff of recalling the past is memories, yet, in the main, very little attention is directed to their examination. Remembering is part and parcel of all our routine daily activities, not just a 'professional activity' of social gerontologists. Yet the pervasiveness of remembering and memories in social life is taken for granted in life history studies. On the whole, how previous events come to be seen as 'memories' is not addressed. When the concept of 'memory' is seen as worthy of comment it tends to be identified as a barrier to reliability and validity, so that researching memory is a technical matter. In this way, too, memory is viewed as a resource in rather than a topic of analysis. Just as Bytheway (1995) has sought to unpack 'age', another bedrock category in the social gerontologist's armoury, so my concern in this chapter is to unravel the category of memories. Put quite simply, my interest is: what are these things called memories? Memories are inevitably and indisputably involved in recalling life, but in the main they are viewed in life histories as a means to an end.

Initially, then, I will examine the analytical and methodological underpinnings of and claims that are made for the study of life histories in the field of ageing. This will enable me to link these claims with the seminal work of G.H. Mead on language usage, the development of the self and memory. Having brought the category of memory to the fore, I want to turn to an exposition of Coulter's ethnomethodological treatment of the category 'memories'. This allows me to differentiate an ethnomethodological approach from that of discursive psychology. It is Coulter's insistence on memories being viewed as a topic for rather than a resource in analysis which promises a different approach to the study of ageing. The novelty of this position will become apparent when I offer a brief analysis of a transcript which features talk about memories. My overall intention in the chapter, then, is to alter the focus on the category memories within the study of ageing, by moving it from a peripheral to a more central line of vision.

## Life histories and ageing

Arguably, studies of the life course have been underpinned by two general theoretical concerns: first, with a broad notion of social change; second, with changes in individual identity throughout life. Such emphases might be viewed as reflecting a conventional sociological interest in macro and micro features of social life.

Concentration on broader notions of social change is evident in Bertaux's (1981) collection of papers. For Bertaux, the biographical method is part of a wider agenda of industrial and structural change. Life histories offer the possibility of making a linkage between the individual and social structure and, particularly, between the individual and general socio-historical changes.

Researchers working within the tradition often acknowledge  their debt to the pioneering work of Thomas and Znaniecki (1958). In doing so, they clearly demonstrate their particular concerns with social change and the individual. Thus, Gagnon (1981) notes that Thomas and Znaniecki's study of the Polish peasant was motivated by the intention of controlling social change through the discovery of the psychological laws governing the process. Similarly, Kohli (1981) argued that Thomas and Znaniecki intended the biographical method to give access to the reality of the life of social aggregates.

This focus on life histories as a means to capture the influence of wider social change on individuals' experience has been identified as an example of historical sociology. Humphrey (1993) refers to Abrams's (1982) advocacy of such an approach as a way of furthering our understanding of 'the puzzle of human agency' through 'the process of social structuring'. As I shall suggest subsequently, though, these distinctions are part of an epistemological framework which obscures rather than clarifies the category of memory/memories.

The focus on change and individual identity in later life is particularly evident in British studies of the life course (Johnson 1976; di Gregorio 1986; Dant and Gearing 1990; Bytheway 1993; Humphrey 1993). Within this approach, the elaboration of individual identity in later life rests upon the concept of career derived from symbolic interactionism. Career is seen as a way of capturing the dynamic, processual features of social life. As individuals move through different phases of their life, the meanings attached to events in them may change and vary. This standpoint is taken to present a specific entrée into studying the life course, for it allows changes in identity experienced throughout life to be pinpointed. In this way current experiences in later life may be understood in terms of past ones.

Though I have noted different approaches to the study of individual experience in life history research, I would suggest that they are characterized by what might be termed 'family resemblances'. While not showing one theoretical approach, they seem to exhibit one specific feature. The adoption of the life history method was a response to dissatisfaction with studies based on a medical model of ageing or reliant upon the social survey as routes to understanding the process of ageing. Such approaches were considered to diminish the primacy of individuals' own experiences and the meanings they themselves attached to them. Often, though not necessarily appropriately, the life history method is advocated as an anti-positivist approach. In this sense, life histories are seen as acting as a counterpoint to previous approaches. The perspective of the individual, his or her own interpretation of events, is the focus of enquiry. In contrast to the survey approach, *a priori* categories of the researcher are avoided and replaced by those of the researched: the individual's own perspective is paramount in the analysis.

A consequence of the attempt to offer a view of ageing which specifically aimed to provide an alternative to structural functionalism, as epitomized in the disengagement thesis, was that the individual's own experience was assigned a privileged status (Silverman 1993). Capturing experience, of itself, was a guarantee of authenticity and, thereby, validity. Silverman's reservations are demonstrated in Humphrey (1993), when he claims that life histories provide rich, qualitative data to describe people's own lives in their own words. Over and above this, Humphrey's (1993) claims have a particular relevance to this chapter, for he explicitly addresses the matter of 'memory'.

> The account's wholeness will rest on the accuracy of memory as past experience can be repressed or merged with others; its reliability will depend in part on the nature of the story the respondent desires to tell which will in turn be influenced by his or her current situation and state of mind.
>
> (Humphrey 1993: 168)

Those studies emphasizing the experience of individuals reflect an epistemological framework based upon a 'correspondence theory of truth'. Indeed, Humphrey specifically refers to the creation of life histories which 'bear adequate correspondence to actual individual life histories' (Humphrey 1993: 169). Davies (1993) has recently addressed these issues in relation to the life history approach. She argues that accounts, resting upon a 'correspondence theory of truth', are taken to stand on behalf of reality and are distinguishable from and have an existence apart from the text. She maintains that such matters involved ideas about 'inner' and 'outer' reality. These distinctions reflect those made earlier to 'human agency' and 'social structure'. In contrast to this framework, Davies advocates an epistemological approach based upon a 'coherence theory of truth', whereby the account is a topic in its own right. It is through culturally available procedures that 'Members constitute the world and in so doing they engage ongoingly and irremediably in the production of social and moral activities' (Davies 1993: 118). It should be emphasized that although matters such as gender and ethnicity are conventionally analysed within a correspondence theory of reality, there is no reason why they cannot be part of a coherence view of reality. The concern would be how gender and ethnicity are constituted in social interaction. Here I intend to pursue the path suggested by Davies.

## Objects and memories in Mead

Symbolic interactionism, to which earlier reference has been made, had its intellectual roots in the philosophy of G.H. Mead (1934), though he himself never used the term. Mind, for Mead, while including the idea of a biological organism, was more than that: it was overwhelmingly a social phenomenon. Out of our participation in social groups grows individual behaviour and experience. This activity involves the use of language, which, for Mead, encompassed a story of 'significant symbols'. Such 'significant symbols' were called upon and were crucial in Mead's perspective on the development of mind and self. It was through language that recognizing and taking the role of the 'generalized other' was possible, and consequently 'I', 'me' and 'self' could be developed. Though Mead assigned a central place to language in his philosophy, in that social phenomena were linguistically constructed, many contemporary adherents of symbolic interactionism have neglected his concern with language (Watson 1994). While this comment was not originally made with specific reference to studies of the life course, it is, nevertheless, apposite to them, for, as has been noted already, many employ a symbolic interactionist framework.

For Mead, it was through language that ordinary material objects, such as chairs and tables, are constituted. It is in such socially organized matters that the uses to which objects should be put arise, rather than residing in some notion of their intrinsic physical properties. The object, then, may be conceptualized as generating lists of instructions about how to act towards it. Mead's insistence on behaviour emanating from orientation to a 'generalized other' extended to picturing objects in this way, as well as individuals. Since Mead (1938) emphasized the social nature of the mind and self being dependent upon the absorption of others' experience with our own, it is not surprising that his treatment of memories followed a similar path. The inevitability of taking others' experience into account is that individuals attach the same validity to those experiences as to their own. Again the role of language is crucial here. For Mead, 'memory images' are 'refreshed' and built up through the mechanism of language. It is through conversations which relate social experience that the past is expressed.

While Mead displays a thoroughly sociological dimension to the study of objects and memories, the unproblematic status assigned to experience rather limits how we might examine these matters in social situations. Coulter suggests a way out of this impasse and it is to his work that we may now turn.

## Coulter on memory

Coulter has written extensively on sociological approaches to the study of psychological phenomena. In particular, he considers memory in terms of 'the socially organised character of recollection and forgetting' (Coulter 1979: 59). Although he clearly does not dissent from Mead's position that memories are social phenomena, Coulter eschews Mead's qualifications of memory in terms of 'memory record' and 'memory image', for he emphasizes that the public display of memory is a socially organized accomplishment evident in talk and reliant upon cultural knowledge. So, while allocating a central place to language, just as Mead does, he also adds a specific focus on individuals' use of cultural knowledge. A pivotal feature of Coulter's treatment of memory is that 'remembering is a defeasible achievement and not purely a mental process' (Coulter 1979: 59). By defeasible Coulter means that remembering is defined through exception rather than necessary and sufficient conditions, whether they be physical or psychological. Hence, remembering and forgetting go together. Moreover, the former is not a state or an event. That remembering is a defeasible accomplishment is evident when, upon being asked to recall something, we select from an array of knowledge which is conventionally seen as appropriate to the interests of the speaker and the hearer; a matter to which Sacks *et al.* (1974) referred as 'recipient design'.

Coulter goes on to point out that there are some things we are normatively expected to remember and some we are normatively entitled to claim to have forgotten. Hence, forgetting events such as meeting children from school or anniversaries fall into the former category, and are viewed as a moral rather than a cognitive failure. 'Forgetting' a traumatic event is permissible, even if it actually has not been forgotten.

In his later work, Coulter (1991) links a 'storage' view of memory to the Cartesian dualism between mind and body: memories are stored in the mental space of the mind and retrieved by a search process. According to Coulter, materialist philosophers would argue against the Cartesian perspective and for our brains being the location of storage, retrieval and remembering. In this way, memories are depicted as '*themselves* neurally encoded phenomena', but Coulter suggests that we should consider neural structures as a means of

> facilitating *the situated production* of *memory claims* (to oneself or others) in all their variety. Furthermore, by thinking of remembering in this way, the presumed 'gap' between a 'memory' and its 'retrieval' can be seen to be an *artefact* of storage theorizing rather than a genuine puzzle for it to solve.
>
> (Coulter 1991: 188; emphases in the original)

Coulter's comments are pertinent to the concerns of this chapter in at least two ways. First, while he shares Mead's emphasis on language, unlike him, Coulter recognizes implicitly the residual mentalism apparent in Mead's notion of memory images. Second, his approach can account for how the examination of memory as a technical problem relating to 'accuracy' (Humphrey 1993) and recall/truth (Dant and Gearing 1990), and thereby to validity of data (Plummer 1983), is a consequence of a storage view of memory. A crucial matter for Coulter is that all cognitive phenomena, not just memories, are properties of persons and do not themselves have an ontological existence. An ethnomethodological focus on memory treats it 'as embedded within, and, available from, shared communicative and other forms of activities' of persons. A central concern, then, is with how people tell their memories in talk. It is to that matter that we shall subsequently turn.

Before turning to an explicit focus on the ways in which memories are a matter situated in language usage, I need to anticipate and address a possible criticism of my approach. It might be argued that, since my concern and those of Coulter's are shared with discursive psychologists, I am not adding anything new to the study of memory. As I now intend to show, while the problematics of memory are shared, the resolution of them is different.

Psychologists have recently turned their attention to naturally occurring conversational discourse. Discourse analysis entails a focus on naturally occurring situations rather than on inner processes, which have been the traditional concerns of psychologists. Discourse analysis is against mind/memory as a processing mechanism/information processing matter, but rather a matter embedded in language (Harre and Stearns 1995).

Discourse analysis of memory has been outlined by Edwards and Potter (1992). Ostensibly their critique of psychological approaches to the study of memory and their proposed solution are not dissimilar to Coulter's. Like him, they point to the limitations of conceptualizing memory in terms of mental constructs, representations and processes. They attempt to locate memory in talk and text as interactional work; to demonstrate how remembering is appropriately understood as situated versions of past events and how versions of the past are accepted as fact. Despite this and their emphasis on naturally occurring events, their reliance on what they call the 'discursive action model' sharply separates Edwards and Potter from Coulter's standpoint. This is not the place to detail this discursive action model, but suffice it to say that it appears *a priori* to list a collection of relevancies for the analysis of memories. Furthermore, they verge on necessary and sufficient conditions required for attaining analysis. This runs counter to Coulter's demonstration that memories are a defeasible achievement. In addition, Edwards and Potter's insistence on remembering/recollecting as an action is problematic. As Coulter (1979: 38) points out, memories do not result from action but are an outcome: we cannot be told to remember but only to try to remember.

## Objects, memories and the life course

Up to now I have examined how memory has been handled in life histories and noted the intellectual connections with Mead. I turned to him because he promised an analysis of memory and objects which was ineluctably social, but to make that evident in language I have called upon Coulter's suggestions. Now I can begin to sketch out how we might make memory more of a central concern in the study of the life course. In elaborating my position that memories are socially organized, I want to show how recollections are publicly displayed through talk about objects. In doing this I want to offer a brief analysis of some data extracts where talk about 'memories' is apparent.

These demonstrate Sacks's (1995) point that memories are 'touched off/triggered off' in interaction. The relevance of this to the life history method is clear here. The very matter of being asked to talk about memories triggers our memories. Just as postmodernists would argue that there is never one life recounted in an autobiography, so I would suggest that the life history method cannot guarantee to lay bare one authentic life based upon experience.

1 . . . But I must admit I don't want to go. It's part
2 of your life you know . . . three children born here, so many memories for me. Still
3 you've got to progress with the times haven't you? . . . What are you going to do
4 with all your things? The things I've got over the years. They're not just material
5 possessions. They're memories. My sister went to live next door. She died. I've
6 got things she bought me, what the children have bought over the years. My
7 collection of Toby jugs which has taken me years. There's more in there. What am
8 I going to do with those things? Things I've brought back from holiday as souvenirs.
9 I can't just throw memories away. So this is a problem.

10 INT: If there was anything you wouldn't part with, what would it be?

11 Well things the children have bought me over the years. The things I've brought back
12 from holidays. As I say, my sister that died, next door, I've a couple of her things.
13 She's been dead years. She was only 29 but I wouldn't, you know. Plus there's
14 Jim's mother. She had some lovely things. I've got some plates. Now they're over
15 a hundred years old, one of them's a meat plate. And she used to say to me, 'Never
16 part with those'. And I wouldn't. She's got two brass candle sticks. Well things
17 like that. I've still got the plates in there because I've got nowhere to put them but
18 what would I do with them? I've promised her I'll never part with them. There's
19 two wall plates in there. Now one of the lads has always wanted them since his gran
20 died so I gave them to him, so that's one problem solved. I've given one of the big
21 plates to one of my daughters-in-law because she collects plates but there's so many
22 other things. There's all my Ruby Wedding things, my Silver Wedding things. Gosh
23 I just don't know what I'm going to do with it all. I won't give it away and yet I
24 don't want to keep them packed up in boxes because I think if you've got nice things
25 you should use them for whatever purpose they're meant. If they're for display,
26 display them. I'm not one for shoving things in a cupboard and only using them
27 when you've got company. I don't know . . . I've stopped getting Toby jugs. Before
28 Christmas I said to Jim, I said, 'I'll just have to get rid of all these Toby jugs.' And
29 he said, 'You can't do that.' He said, 'All them years and the way you've treasured
30 them.' And he's bought me one and my daughter-in-law bought me one and a lot of
31 them are Royal Doulton ones. You couldn't get rid of them. They mean as much
32 to me as the ones that are worth quite some money. I mean that one there – Sir
33 Francis Drake – well I paid £31 for that years ago. That one at the top, King Lear,
34 I paid £20 for that about three years ago at an antiques fair. But you see two of them
35 had bought me Toby jugs for Christmas. I used to love going to antiques fairs. Have
36 you ever been to Charnock Richard? They have an antique fair there, brilliant it is,
37 every Sunday. And I used to go and I used to love it. But you see now I've stopped
38 going because I thought, well what am I going to do with it. Then when I said I was
39 going to get rid of them he went mad. Then I found out he'd bought me that
40 cricketer and one of my daughters-in-law had bought me another one. It's not in
41 there. It's in the other cabinet. But you see a few of those I've bought on holiday.

42 That one of Francis Drake I bought in the Lake District. That one of King Lear was
43 somewhere near Blackpool, at an antique fair there. That one, that Charles Dickens
44 thing, I bought that in Ilfracombe. So everyone, you know. That one down there,
45 that big one, is a musical one. I bought that in Torquay. That was the first one I
46 ever bought.

A reading of these data shows how objects serve as an agenda and are part of the reviewing of life prompted by an intended move to sheltered housing. Moreover, this review of life involves the moral evaluation of objects as memories. In lines 1–3 life is embodied in the house/in memories and particular significant events which occurred there.

From then onwards, the category of memories is elaborated and more importantly publicly made available to us through talk about objects. In lines 4–9 there is a mapping out of which objects may not only constitute memories but how they may be so constituted. In declaring that objects are 'not just material possessions', the common-sense usage of objects as part of an acquisitive, consumerist culture is contested, for those to which reference is made – 'Toby jugs', 'souvenirs' etc. – are frequently cast in this light. In this sense, the Meadian perspective on objects as other than physical matter is evident here.

The dismissal of objects as solely 'material possessions' is followed by the declaration of them as memories. This transformation of objects from the 'material' to the 'memorable' employs cultural knowledge about their origins, which, in turn, convey instructions about their possible fate. 'Presents', as the objects referred to here are implied to be, are different from those which we buy for ourselves (though when we do so we may justify them in terms of a 'treat'). Presents, if not edible, carry the implicit command of 'something to be kept'. Conversely, edible presents, especially chocolates, are to be consumed and, in line with 'good manners', at least offered by the recipient to the giver.

This transformation of objects from the 'material' to the 'memorable' is further amplified by notions about the giver of the present. The closer the relationship of the giver to the recipient, the greater the expectation that the gift should be kept. Here, the givers as 'sister' and 'children' fall under this rubric. This knowledge about objects as presents and their givers underpins that not uncommon practice of ephemerally displaying a present that may not be to our 'taste'. Such considerations, though, are overridden by the source: if it is given by someone 'close' to us, we may display it for the duration of his or her visit to our home.

The constitution of objects as other than 'material' but also as 'memories' points to a dual usage of memories. They are used in the sense of being both object-like and objectified in things, embodied in things. That memories may be object-like is clear in the declaration that they are not to be thrown away. Memories are not disposable but have an enduring quality to them. Such connotations are conveyed in the comment after a death that 'you still have your memories': though the person is not alive, memories of him or her are still alive.

In this sense, too, there is an interesting dialectic between memories as object-like, objectified in things, and persons, the givers of objects. In lines

12–21 mention is made of gifts from deceased persons, a sister and a mother, and as such these gifts are to be kept. In this way, just as memories may be object-like, so may the object serve to personify the memory. Further cultural knowledge about deceased persons in connection with promises informs the retention rather than the disposal of objects. In general, making a promise to someone carries a 'firm' agreement to comply with a request, but not necessarily so: young children may be 'fobbed off' with a promise by parents who have no intention to keep it. The status of the person, then, is of some relevance. Now if the person to whom the promise was made dies, it has a specific moral imperative. Having promised in the past to do something we now will do so, come what may: greater responsibility is assumed for 'keeping the promise'.

The second usage of memories as objectified in things is evident in talk of Toby jugs (lines 27–46). A collection of Toby jugs is specified in terms of previous events in life and the giver. Interestingly, the Toby jugs are personified, given a name of the literary or historical character they represent: King Lear, Sir Francis Drake, Charles Dickens etc. Through the attachment of a particular Toby jug to its giver and place of purchase (often while on holiday), memories are objectified in things.

Memories are not only publicly displayed through talk, they are also and should, as objectified in things, be literally on public display. Objects given at specific events in life, at Silver and Ruby Wedding anniversaries, for instance (lines 22–27), are not only memories for the recipients but are to be shared with others. 'Nice things' are not 'to be shoved [kept] in cupboards "but to be" used for whatever they're meant: if they're for display, display them.' Moreover, by not restricting the use of those objects to 'when you've got company', but by implication making them a part of everyday life, the past becomes part of the present. Paradoxically, then, memories are both past and current matters.

## Concluding remarks

My purpose in this chapter has been to explicate the category of memories and their uses in the life history method. In doing so, I have argued that their place in the recalling of the past, in the telling of a life, has been viewed unproblematically, since the life history method has called upon a correspondence theory of reality. I have shown how British studies of the life course, while often based upon symbolic interactionism, have neglected Mead's emphasis on the role of language in social life. Although his approach links language with memory, his emphasis on memory image reflects a residual mentalism. Despite discursive psychologists' claims to be turning their backs on psychology's traditional 'trait' approach to the study of memory, I argued that their avowedly new approach is limiting. I turned to Coulter's ethnomethodological treatment of cognitive matters, especially memory, to offer a way forward.

I have shown, albeit briefly, how memories are situated in talk about objects when a life is recalled and told. The analysis offered here is far from exhaustive but it should be viewed as an attempt to make a sociological perspective on memories an explicit focus in the study of the life course. In examining the approaches of Mead to objects and memories and Coulter to memory, I have sought to demonstrate that memories need not be employed solely as a resource in analysis and that if, instead, they become a topic for analysis in their own right, they promise a fruitful yield in furthering an understanding of how individuals tell a life.

## Acknowledgements

I should like to acknowledge comments made by Rod Watson on an earlier draft of this paper and to thank Shirley Most for typing.

## References

Abrams, P. (1982) *Historical Sociology*. Shepton Mallet: Open Books.
Bertaux, D. (ed.) (1981) *Biography and Society*. London: Sage.
Bytheway, B. (1993) Ageing and biography: the letter of Bernard and Mary Brenson, *Sociology*, 27(1), 153–65.
Bytheway, B. (1995) *Ageism*. Buckingham: Open University Press.
Coulter, J. (1975) *Approaches to Insanity*. London: Martin Robertson.
Coulter, J. (1979) *The Social Construction of Mind*. London: Macmillan.
Coulter, J. (1991) Cognition: cognition in an ethnomethodological mode, in G. Button (ed.) *Ethnomethodology and the Human Sciences*. Cambridge: Cambridge University Press.
Dant, T. and Gearing, B. (1990) Doing biographical research, in S. Peace (ed.) *Researching Social Gerontology*. London: Sage.
Davies, M. (1993) Healing Sylvia. Accounting for the textual 'discovery' of unconscious knowledge, *Sociology*, 27(1), 160–78.
di Gregorio, S. (1986) Understanding the management of everyday living, in C. Phillipson, M. Bernard and P. Strang (eds) *Dependency and Interdependency in Later Life*. London: Croom-Helm.
Edwards, D. and Potter, J. (1992) *Discursive Psychology*. London: Sage.
Gagnon, N. (1981) On the analysis of life accounts, in D. Bertaux (ed.) *Biography and Society*. London: Sage.
Harre, R. and Stearns, P. (eds) (1995) *Discursive Psychology in Practice*. London: Sage.
Humphrey, R. (1993) Ageing and social life in an ex-mining town, *Sociology*, 27(1), 166–78.
Kohli, M. (1981) Biography: account, text and method, in D. Bertaux (ed.) *Biography and Society*. London: Sage.
Johnson, M. (1976) That was your life: a biographical approach to later life, in J.M.A. Munnichs and W.J.A. Van Den Heuval (eds) *Dependency and Interdependency in Old Age*. The Hague: Nijhoff.
Mead, G.H. (1934) *Mind, Self and Society*. Chicago: University of Chicago Press.
Mead, G.H. (1938) *The Philosophy of the Act*. Chicago: University of Chicago Press.
Plummer, K. (1983) *Documents of Life: an Introduction to the Problems and Literature of a Humanistic Method*. London: Allen & Unwin.
Sacks, H. (1995) *Lectures on Conversations*. Oxford: Blackwell.
Sacks, H., Schegloff, E. and Jefferson, G. (1974) A simplest systematic for the organisation of turn taking for conversation, *Language*, 50, 696–735.

Silverman, D. (1993) *Interpreting Qualitative Data*. London: Sage.
Thomas, W.I. and Znaniecki, F. (1958) *The Polish Peasant in Europe and America*. New York: Dove.
Watson, R. (1994) Symbolic interactionism, in J. Ostman (ed.) *Handbook of Pragmatics*. Amsterdam: John Benjamins.

**PART II**

---

# Conceptualizing age relations and later life

---

**7** MARGOT JEFFERYS

# Inter-generational relationships: an autobiographical perspective

## Introduction

There are three kinds of inter-generational relationships I want to consider from the viewpoint of an older person, adopting broadly a 'life course' perspective. I start with the assumption that earlier experiences from childhood onwards, in both the domestic and work spheres, set the stage and help to determine the kind of relationships which older people have with younger people (Hareven and Adam 1982: xi–xvi; Fennell *et al.* 1988: 49–54; Bond *et al.* 1993: 31–40).

In line with this perspective, the reflections will be autobiographical (Johnson 1978: 99–115; Starr 1982: 255–70; Munnichs 1992: 244–50). The features of my past which I believe were formative in determining my perceptions of my present inter-generational relationships are largely structural. By that I mean that they consisted of the general social, cultural and economic conditions which I have shared throughout my life with those of my contemporaries who were born into relatively affluent, stable British middle-class families in the early years of the twentieth century. For this reason, I expect the account, including the meanings I attach to relationships, to have some degree of generalizability and an explanatory value beyond the purely personal.

This is not to argue, however, that other factors, including genetic endowment and idiosyncratic personality characteristics, play no part in the way my current relationships with younger people are shaped and the meanings that I attach to them. No other individual, even of the same gender and social class, reared in roughly comparable circumstances and exposed to approximately the same experiences, would have had exactly the same reaction to them. In these reflections, therefore, I try to estimate the extent to which my inter-generational relationships today and my feelings about them are likely to be more or less representative of those of my own peer group, and, if they are not, the kind of factors which could account for possible variations.

Adopting a 'life course' perspective also implies a commitment to a view of ageing which places the emphasis on the peculiar if not unique social, economic and cultural features of the specific historical period in which the concomitant, inevitable biological ageing process takes place (Dannefer and Sell 1988). To that extent, I endorse the proposition that 'ageing' is a social construct. At the same time, I am very much aware of the self – my self – as an embodied entity experiencing diminishing physical capability and mental agility. These realities contribute to parallel changes in inclinations and motivations to undertake once-cherished activities. Hence, I do not propose to deny the reality of biological ageing, the course of which itself is likely to be the combined outcome of genetic endowment and the myriad positive and negative influences of events and circumstances through 80 years of existence (Black 1988: 163–5; Featherstone and Hepworth 1991).

The three kinds of inter-generational relationships I consider are those I have with (a) middle-aged offspring, (b) grown-up grandchildren and (c) past and present younger work colleagues.

In selecting which topics to give special consideration to in each type of relationship, I have been influenced by the dominant themes in the burgeoning social gerontological literature, as well as by the manifestations of popular media interest in 'problematic' aspects of inter-generational relationships. These include such issues as 'the generation gap', 'equity', 'reciprocity' and the 'burden' of an ageing population on the rest of society. To some extent, I have pitted my own experience against both sociological theories and the findings of empirical studies. In some cases, there is a good match; in other cases, my own experience seems to depart to some extent from one or the other.

## The individual and the changing social context

Some biographical details will serve to place me in a recognizable social context. I am now in my eightieth year and, along with a majority of my birth cohort, have lived much longer than the expectation of life of females at the time of my birth (which was roughly 57 years). The majority of those of us who have survived thus far can expect to live at least another eight years (Government Actuary 1992). These stark survival statistics indicate that I was a member of a cohort whose expectation of life increased as mortality declined dramatically. (In parenthesis, perhaps this extraordinary change accounts for some of the widespread belief in my generation that human progress is 'natural' and set-backs are 'unnatural'.) The decline in mortality itself was the combined result of improved nutrition, prophylactic public health measures which reduced the prevalence and/or severity of infectious diseases of childhood, adolescence and early adult life, and safer and less frequent child-bearing. My contemporaries are also apt to attribute the decline to clinical and surgical advances, 'the miracles of modern medicine', although these latter played only a small part until the past two decades (McKeown 1976).

Subsequent birth cohorts have also seen improvements in their longevity during their lifetimes, but at a rather slower pace. Mortality rates of those who have already passed the rubicon of three score years and ten, however, continue to fall. Less certain is whether longer life is or is not accompanied by a better quality of life or less disability (Manton and Stallard 1994; Bone 1995; Dunnell 1995).

I was one of four siblings, a fairly typical family size for the period. Both my parents' backgrounds were professional, comparatively well-to-do economically, and above all secure in public sector or non-commercial, usually tenured, jobs. In the inter-war years, I went to a private school, followed by university. The latter was still an unusual pathway for even middle-class girls to follow. Despite their reduced chances of success in the matrimonial stakes, given the contemporary surplus of women of child-bearing age, they were still most likely to assume that early marriage was the only desirable and legitimate career aim. Except in very limited instances, it was not possible to combine it with professional work.

I was in my early twenties when the Second World War broke out. Virtually overnight, attitudes to married women working changed. I abandoned postgraduate work and, after marrying in 1941, worked in the Midlands in various factory and other jobs requiring no skills or training. Most of my university colleagues went into managerial or civil service posts. I became pregnant in 1943 and had two children with only a short interval between them, by which time the war was over and I returned with my new family to London (Jefferys 1978: 135–61).

After the war, some of my friends were influenced by the prevailing postwar social pressure on women to retreat from paid employment to the domestic sphere. The pressure was reinforced by the work of Bowlby (1965), which was widely interpreted as meaning that infants would be psychologically damaged if they were deprived of the full-time attention of their mothers. I, however, was not willing to yield to these pressures and never gave up work outside the home entirely, although initially it was part-time and sporadic. When my younger son was 18 months old, I was fortunate to find an unmarried mother living nearby who acted as mother substitute and domestic help for the following 12 years, giving continuity of child care until my sons were well into their teens. This was unusually serendipitous. Some of my peer group experienced a range of difficulties (for example, in accommodating a succession of au pair girls) which I did not have to face.

My own full-time career from my thirties onwards was as an academic teacher and researcher, always in the London area. My marriage began to fall apart in the mid-1950s. It ended formally in divorce when I was 40 and our sons were in their early teens. Lone parenthood was less common in the 1950s and 1960s than it is today (Coleman 1988: 61–9). I believe my sons were sensitively aware that I was 'different' from most of their peer group's mothers and didn't like it. Because I was in a tenured reasonably paid post, the consequence of the break-up was far less crippling financially than that suffered by many other lone mothers both at the time and since. I was also cushioned, unlike many others, from the unavoidable emotional trauma by an absorbing job, supportive work colleagues and an extensive network of good friends. Nevertheless, the whole experience was painful and may well have had a greater influence on my subsequent life and on my relationships with my offspring and grandchildren than I have so far been able to acknowledge.

This brief biographical sketch, I hope, will help to set my present intergenerational relationships in a historical context. It is also suggestive of the factors that may account for the characteristics of those relationships which may not be typical of those of my age and gender peers.

## Relationships with middle-aged children

Much of the literature dealing with the nature and quality of relationships between parents and their middle-aged children has focused on the extent to which contact between them has been maintained in the first place, and on the purpose(s), nature and quality of the contact. Interest has focused on the kind of instrumental and affective support tasks which are performed and the extent to which they depend upon such factors as the genders of the parental survivor and of the middle-aged offspring, or on the number, geographical location and availability of the latter (Shanas *et al.* 1965; Gubrium 1976). Many studies have been predicated on the assumption that the older person, particularly if widowed, is dependent, and the recipient rather than the donor of affective support as well as instrumental services (Phillipson 1991). Some, however, have been aware of the inherent bias in studies based primarily on the experience of those who have, for one reason or another, come to the attention of health or welfare services. Studies which have disaggregated the single category of 'old age', covering all those who have reached the statutory retirement age, have indicated that dependency needs increase at an accelerating pace with advancing age (Hunt 1978). Others have shown that the great majority of retired people in industrialized societies today defy the stereotypes of old age as a period of inevitable decrepitude. 'Old age' is marked by as great a variability in health experiences and in lifestyles as is an equivalent number of years of middle life (Black 1985).

My own experience suggests that the nature of my present relationships with my middle-aged offspring is the outcome of a number of factors, including, significantly, the level of my present dependency needs, which are likely to change if I survive much longer, perhaps drastically. At present, there are first some internalized assumptions about how we should behave towards one another. I believe that for the most part we share these assumptions (which, I believe, do most others of our two generations). They include, basically, the assumption that each generation's primary obligation is to its own descendant dependents, and that we do not offer each other gratuitous advice on how it should be performed. Then there are the affectional ties developed over a lifetime: in our case they are very strong.

My face-to-face contacts with my two sons and their wives are irregular. The occasions on which we meet habitually include birthdays and annual holiday periods such as Christmas; otherwise meeting depends mainly on the chance convenience of 'fitting in' visits with other social commitments. Although I live within a few minutes' drive of one son's family and occasionally drop in on my way home from work or shopping, contact with both sons is generally by telephone, initiated by me. There is, I believe, a tacit agreement that the 'work' involved in ensuring the continuity and quality of the relationship at present appropriately devolves on me because they have less time to invest in relationship maintenance and less intrinsic reward from doing so than me. In all these ways, my experience seems typical of that experienced by my peer group (Jerrome 1993).

As I have so far been able to obtain paid help with my housework and gardening, and have had no major health problems requiring help with nursing or personal hygiene, I have not needed to ask kin for help with activities of daily living. However, in the past ten years or so I have come to rely on one of my sons to advise me on my income tax returns and on how to manage my financial affairs. I count this an invaluable service, since it saves me the time and energy I would otherwise need either to undertake this disagreeable task myself or to seek out a reliable commercial advisor to do it for me. An added attraction of having these affairs overseen for me by a son is the satisfaction derived from believing that the decisions are such that my personal financial resources are in many respects taking on the form of 'extended family resources'. I like the feeling that they are being used at one and the same time to ensure as far as possible that I shall not experience indignities purely on account of lack of money if or as I require more support, while providing grandchildren with some welcome financial help now, when they have only limited resources but expanding needs and desires for independence. I call on my other son to help me resolve technical problems associated with word-processing and data management.

Given my relatively good health, independence in the activities of daily living and financial ease, it is not surprising that the concept of constituting a 'burden' on my sons has not so far seemed relevant to me, or, I hope, to them. Nor, thanks to their own economic situations, have I had to consider supporting them financially, as some of my contemporaries have had to do for their less fortunate offspring, some of whom have unexpectedly had to face unemployment in middle age (Binney and Estes 1988). Perhaps my continuing commitment to various academic-type pursuits has also spared them from any inclination I might have had to offer them gratuitous advice on their affairs.

As to the indeterminate future, I am totally confident that, if or when I become physically or mentally frail and am no longer able to function with reasonable dignity on my own, I shall be able to rely on both sons and their spouses to make decisions for me, and see to it that I live and die as comfortably as possible. As a result, I do not live in dread of a future loss of autonomy. I think I shall be quite happy to yield it up to them, if and when 'the time comes'. I cannot think of any greater traumatic experience that I could suffer than that any one of them, their spouses or children should die or suffer a serious misfortune while I am still alive.

## Grandchildren

The sociological literature on grandparenting has burgeoned in the past decade. Earlier studies of the family in industrial society had suggested that, although more people were surviving long enough to become grandparents, other features of the economy – greater geographical labour mobility and the reduction in multi-generational households – together with smaller family size, operated to reduce the part played by older women, in particular, in supporting their daughters or daughters-in-law in their child-rearing activities (Young and Willmott 1957).

Nevertheless, recent studies based on empirical data suggest that grandparenthood remains a welcomed status. It helps to compensate for the more disagreeable aspects of ageing. Even if, in current times, contributing to the household and child-rearing tasks may be less important aspects of the role for many grandparents, affectional bonds forged between them and their grandchildren help to sustain the cohesion of the family as a primary socializing unit, while providing immediate gratification to all concerned (Albrecht 1954).

At the same time, other studies have indicated that the euphoric idyllic picture of grandparenting – often portrayed in TV advertisements – could conceal tensions, the downside of the relationship. For example, there could be conflict between parents and grandparents about how to 'bring up' young children, and mutual accusations of 'spoiling', still regarded by some as a heinous crime (Thompson *et al.* 1990).

Some of the contributors to an important volume of essays on grandparenthood (Bengtson and Robertson 1985) linked the phenomenon with the issue of what has come to be encapsulated in the term 'generation gap'. For example, Gutman (1985) suggested that grandparenting was not a satisfying role for many older Americans today. He attributed this to values being much at variance between generations. Contemporary society, he alleged, was brash and materialistic compared with the one in which he had been reared. The present younger generation had been socialized into believing that 'young is beautiful, old is ugly' in metaphorical as well as descriptive terms.

Does my own experience of grandparenthood match up to any of these sociological approaches to the status and its corresponding role?

I certainly had a great desire to become a grandmother. It was almost as compelling and intense as my earlier desire to be a mother. I cannot rule out the possibility that both urges were due to some perception that the statuses would give me added social standing as well as a sense of achievement. I remember feeling proud that I had become a grandmother before some of my same age peers. It was almost a competitive game. I don't think, however, that I was motivated by the feeling that grandparenting would compensate me for what are often regarded as mid-life losses; for example, the 'empty nest' syndrome, the breakdown of the marriage partnership, the menopause and libido decline. My professional and social life at the time was satisfying and full, and my health excellent. But who is to say?

The satisfaction derived from my actual relationships with my six grandchildren collectively and individually has changed with time. When they were very young – babies, infants and primary school age – I had intense pleasure whenever I saw them, and felt it was reciprocated. However, I played no significant part in caring for them then or later. Our contacts were always episodic and irregular.

When they reached puberty and adolescence, they showed less spontaneous pleasure when seeing me than they had earlier in life. We did not develop the close ties based on exchange of confidences which have been the stuff of some other grandparental anecdotal reminiscences (Thompson *et al.* 1990: 174–212). We did not discuss events or ideas which mattered to them. They seemed positively to avoid topics relating to their future career or leisure plans, even when my experience or network of friends and colleagues might have had something to offer them. They seemed afraid of developing any sense of obligation to me.

I attributed their reluctance and the distancing during adolescence – a distancing which always differed somewhat between individual members of the two families, to which I have not done justice and which, in any case, began to diminish as they reached their twenties – to a number of factors. Some of these I believe to be very general; that is, a common feature of the relationships between kin in these two specific twentieth-century birth cohorts. Others I think are more idiosyncratic, related to my particular social circumstances and personal characteristics.

I sent copies of an earlier draft of this chapter to each of my grandchildren and to their parents. The responses it elicited from members of both families – particularly concerning my perceptions of the reasons for the uneasiness in my relationships with my granddaughters – reinforced some of the explanatory propositions I made but undermined others. What follows reflects, therefore, not only my initial thoughts but also the modifications I want to make in them in the light of the feedback I have had from my children and some of my grandchildren.

In my first draft, I wrote of the disappointment, which I believed was shared by many of my contemporaries, when the gifts – particularly sizeable sums of money – I enjoyed giving did not get much response even in the way of acknowledgement, let alone expressions of gratitude. I suggested possible reasons for our erroneous expectations and hence inevitable disappointment. I instanced, for example, the change which had occurred in 50 or 60 years in the value of money, and the growing access of young people to facilities and their ownership of goods which were once regarded as luxuries. I pointed out that my generation has had trouble in coming to terms with the fall in the value of the pound sterling. Sums which still seem large to us could seem relatively insignificant to a younger generation. The fall in the value of money which the older but not the younger generation has witnessed could have come to symbolize for my contemporaries a general feeling of an insecure world of change, where many of the assumptions we made about human behaviours and values could no longer be taken for granted.

For example, there had been some security in the conventional pressures to which we but certainly not our grandchildren had been subjected in childhood, to be deferential to our elders and to acknowledge punctually and politely any gifts we might receive from them. I recognized that, in the light of the present global insecurities, the young may well feel ambivalent to say the least about the legacy left them by my generation and certainly no special sense of obligation. They cannot be blamed for cynicism about the motives of establishment figures in every walk of life. In so far as older kin are themselves seen as authority figures, they cannot expect to acquire automatic respect.

In the same vein, my age peers may be less sensitive to the use of kin and personal friendship networks to promote job prospects than those at present in their twenties. The latter, although they belong to a generation demonstrably less engaged in party political matters, are probably more intrinsically egalitarian. Certainly, one of my granddaughters emphasized to me that she had been brought up to feel that it was wrong to use family connections to obtain particular consideration for jobs or other privileges. She wanted to succeed on her own merits rather than owe anything to being the granddaughter of someone with a title which conferred status – at least in the academic world.

One of my sons felt that my draft, despite its efforts at explanation rather than condemnation of the grandchildren, was still unfair on them, and that I had mistaken informality of communication style for indifference and lack of gratitude. A granddaughter pointed out that not until she went to university did she appreciate the money gifts, which previously had been banked rather than spent. She had not seen them as tokens of love or affection, requiring a reciprocal gesture. I had to ask myself, 'Why should she have done?' To her my gifts of books or souvenirs acquired on overseas trips were more meaningful. I think she and her contemporaries, however, are unaware of the diffidence which persuades many grandparents to give spending money rather than gifts which they fear may be rejected – given the observable changes in cultural norms and preferences. This could lead to what she described as 'crossed wires'.

In my first draft I contrasted what I believed to be a much closer relationship between my grandchildren and their maternal grandmothers than between them and me, and suggested that this might account for the lack of intimacy. I pointed out that this was consistent with sociological theories and empirical findings which showed that in countries with a Western Judaeo-Christian heritage mother–adult daughter relationships were on the whole closer and more enduring than mother–adult son relationships. That relationship was cemented by the rendering of essentially domestic reciprocal services feasible in an essentially matrilocal pattern of habitation. I even went on to speculate as to whether this was evidence of the biological advantaging of adult female bonding because it assisted the preservation of the species!

In retrospect, and in the light of comments from my own offspring, I need to make a more than partial if not a total retraction of my causal hypothesis. In so far as it was acknowledged that they had been 'closer' to their maternal grandmother during their teens than to me – and this assertion itself was not totally acceptable to all of them – they refused to attribute it to any fundamental enduring quality of mother–daughter relationships *per se*. Rather, they considered it to be mainly a function of the effect on their perceptions of the meaning to them of their grandmothers' very different life foci.

In contrast to both the maternal grandmothers, I was in full-time, all-absorbing academic, work throughout their childhood and adolescence, and indeed into their early adult life. Not only did this mean that I was unavailable to take on any regular child-rearing chores or special treats even if their mothers had wanted me to. It also meant that my grandchildren gained a view of me as someone who was more interested in my work and the social life surrounding it than I was in family concerns.

Furthermore, because they had internalized the values of a milieu in which academic success was treated with particular respect, all my grandchildren may have been somewhat in awe of me, a feeling which could overlay responses to me on a more personal level. One grandchild, responding to the first draft of this chapter, gave me a fresh insight into our relationships when she wrote frankly:

> I think the main point here is, for me at least, I found you (and still do to some extent) an intimidating person. I spent most of the time in your company worried about how my behaviour, dress and ability to speak was being compared to the cousins (twins) who seemed like angels in comparison. I think I felt stupid (I still suffer from a feeling of intellectual inferiority based on never being able academically to compete with previous family members, mum, dad, you and James [her paternal grandfather] . . . I think that children are not given enough confidence to express themselves intellectually (it's looked down upon in young people's groups) and I think this lack of confidence was increased in your company as you seemed to generate an air of certitude and knowledge which was extremely intimidating. Plus 'discussions' tended to feel like interrogations as you have quite an aggressive manner in conversations. I still feel intimidated intellectually in your company but this has been decreasing over the last few years, and I enjoy being able to talk to you about topics that crop up while I'm visiting.

I find this analysis a very persuasive one. It does not follow, of course, that 'intellectuals' are always likely to be at some disadvantage in bonding with their grandchildren compared with others of their generation. I have also to consider particular personality traits. I think, for example, that I never acquired the lightness of touch and humour which might have seduced them more effectively into exciting and satisfying dialogue. Like some of Thompson et al.'s (1990) grandparents, therefore, I don't believe I played a significant part in their emotional or intellectual development at any stage of their lives, and I am sad that this should have been so.

These explanations for the shortcomings in my experiences of grandparenting compared with my rosy expectations of the role and its contingent relationships have required a degree of self-examination which I normally would not undertake. It has also, I realize, hazarded my relationship with descendant kin. As a natural optimist, however, I hope that the exercise has not been too painful for all those personally involved in it. Indeed, I hope it has ultimately helped to sustain and improve relationships.

I suspect that grandparenting for many of my generation has not always lived up to our idyllic expectations when we were launched only too willingly into the role. Tensions are likely to be ubiquitous facets of the inescapable replacement of one generation by another. The exact character of the tensions, on the other hand, and the way in which they are handled, are much more likely to be determined by family structures and conventions, by the specific life courses of members of all the generations involved and by the pressures exerted by wider social and economic change (Gubrium 1976).

## Work colleagues

As this narrative has already shown, my work was a central source of life satisfaction for me. This was owing equally to its intrinsic content and to the social environment provided by congenial colleagues and eager students in the academic institutions where I worked.

I had had security of tenure until the end of the academic year in which my sixty-fifth birthday fell. I did not welcome compulsory retirement, fearing that with it I would lose my sense of purpose and consequently my self-esteem. In the event, for several reasons, my fears proved unwarranted. Since my formal retirement I have been invited to participate in a variety of part- and full-time consultancies and, quite recently, given the academic respectability and generous privileges of an honorary professorship in a university department. As a result, I can make and maintain contact with academics from several social science disciplines in the field of social gerontology, and have developed close contacts with some lawyers and philosophers interested in health service problematics. They have widened my horizons and given me a new interest in seeing how far our disciplines have things to offer each other. In short, there has been a continuity between my pre- and post-retirement professional life. I feel I continue to belong to a significant movement devoted to valuable intellectual pursuits.

Nevertheless, my personal relationships with both past and present colleagues are somewhat different from those I once had with working colleagues. For example, I am now aware of a degree of deference paid me, which I ascribe to my age. In one sense this is gratifying, but in another it seems a distancing device, telling me that I am understandably no longer quite 'one of them'. Not surprisingly, I sometimes wonder whether protestations of the value of my continuing contribution are essentially token gestures, reflecting either genuine personal affection or a politically correct anti-ageist stance.

I realize too how many changes have occurred in the 14 years since I received an occupational pension. Those years have witnessed, for example, a staggering, virtually exponential change in the technology available to those engaged in research and/or scholarship in the social sciences. Those still engaged in the formal academic and professional labour market have had to acquire a new range of skills simply to maintain their credibility as teachers, researchers and authors. Moreover, they are living in a time of tumultuous and often bitterly resented change in the previously predictable and secure academic world. Now they are uncertain about the present and future, alien management procedures and an ambience which appears to offer nothing but stressful constant judgemental assessments of performance.

Whether or not those of us who are no longer gainfully employed retain an active interest in our academic fields, we are not subject to these last, often unwelcome, pressures. We often express thankfulness at being out of the 'rat race', and we congratulate ourselves on having experienced our working lives in a golden expansionist era in academia. We do not envy our successors.

Those of us who wish to continue to operate in the field as independent, self-employed, self-motivated activists are aware of pressures in a rather different form and with a rather different intensity. To make any significant contribution we have, at the very least, to have access to the new information technology and master it sufficiently to know what it can and cannot provide for us.

Some of my contemporaries have not wanted to meet this challenge. They have quit and chosen new pursuits. Some have had no regrets in leaving, others have found it depressing and hanker after their old activities. Others, like me, have tried to keep their end up. The real rewards have probably been as much the maintenance of meaningful social ties with colleagues of all ages as they have been continued academic achievement or recognition. Yet I suspect that, from time to time, we all ask ourselves whether the physical and mental effort involved and the self-imposed pressures to perform (at a time when our bodies if not our minds are more subject to fatigue) are worth the candle. For many others of my generation, pensioned relatively affluent retirement has been an opportunity to develop interests, pursuits and friendships which were formerly restricted by work commitments.

## Some general reflections

These reflections on how far my personal experience of certain kinds of inter-generational relationships resonates with the general thrust of relevant sociological perspectives on ageing has, on the whole, given me confidence in their strength.

When I agreed to contribute to this book, I was by no means certain whether the received current sociological orthodoxies would help me to understand and structure my experience and illuminate my personal life trajectory. On the whole, I found much in the literature which was confirmatory. When it did not match I could usually find satisfactory explanations for differences. Somewhat disappointingly, I did not find myself wanting to draw attention to new dimensions of actual phenomena, perceptions and meanings relating to inter-generational relationships which had not been adequately addressed.

What I am less clear about is whether my account of the general socio-historical as well as the specific historico-biographical contexts in which my personal inter-generational relationships were embedded are likely to have anything other than anecdotal or illustrative value. It is a question which, for me, still hangs unresolved over the nature of the contribution which oral history provides to our more general understanding of the social world, in which age and ageing as a social process are now beginning to receive overdue consideration.

## References

Albrecht, R. (1954) The parental responsibilities of grandparents, *Marriage and Family Living*, xvi(3), 201–4.

Bengtson, V.L. and Robertson, J.F. (eds) (1985) *Grandparenthood*. Beverly Hills, CA: Sage.

Binney, E. and Estes, C. (1988) The retreat of the state and its transfer of responsibility, *International Journal of Health Services*, 18(1), 83–96.

Black, N. (ed. in chief) (1985) *Birth to Old Age*. Milton Keynes: Open University Press.

Bond, J., Coleman, P. and Peace, S. (eds) (1993) *Ageing in Society*. London: Sage.

Bone, M. (ed.) (1995) *Health Expectancy and Its Uses*. London: HMSO.

Bowlby, J. (1965) *Child Care and the Growth of Love*, 2nd edn. Harmondsworth: Penguin.

Coleman, D.A. (1988) 'Population', in A.H. Halsey (ed.) *British Social Trends since 1900*. Basingstoke: Macmillan.

Cotterill, P. (1994) *Friendly Relations? Mothers and Daughters-in-law*. Basingstoke: Taylor & Francis.

Dannefer, D. and Sell, R.R. (1988) Age structure, the life course transitions and 'aged heterogeneity': prospects for research and theory, *Comprehensive Gerontology*, 1, 1–10.

Dunnell, K. (1995) Are we healthier?, *Population Trends*, 82. London: HMSO.

Featherstone, M. and Hepworth, M. (1991) The mask of aging and the post-modern life course, in M. Featherstone, M. Hepworth and B.S. Turner (eds) *The Body: Social Process and Cultural Theory*. London: Sage.

Fennell, G., Phillipson, C. and Evers, H. (1988) *The Sociology of Old Age*. Milton Keynes: Open University Press.

Government Actuary (1992) *Life Tables. Mortality Statistics. General*. London: HMSO.

Gubrium, J.F. (1976) *Time, Role and Self in Old Age*. New York: Human Sciences Press.

Gutman, D.L. (1985) American origins: the repudiation of gerontocracy, in V.L. Bengtson and J.L. Robertson (eds) *Grandparenthood*. Beverly Hills, CA: Sage, 173–81.

Hareven, T.K. and Adam, K.J. (1982) *Aging and Life Course Transitions: an Interdisciplinary Perspective*. London: Tavistock.

Hunt, A. (1978) The elderly: age difference in the quality of life, *Population Trends*, Spring, 10–16.

Jefferys, M. (1978) Serendipity: an autobiographical account of the career of a medical sociologist in Britain, in R.H. Elling and M. Sokolowska (eds) *Medical Sociologists at Work*. New Brunswick, NJ: Transactions Books.

Jerrome, D. (1993) Intimate relationships, in J. Bond, P. Coleman and S. Peace (eds) *Ageing in Society*, 2nd edn. London: Sage, 237–40.

Johnson, M. (1978) That was your life: a biographical approach to later life, in V. Carver and P. Liddiard (eds) *An Ageing Population*. Sevenoaks: Hodder & Stoughton, 99–115.

Lancaster, J.B. (1985) Evolutionary prospectives on sex differences in the higher primates, in A.S. Rossi (ed.) *Gender and the Life Course*. New York: Aldine, 3–28.

McKeown, T. (1976) *The Role Of Medicine. Dream, Mirage or Nemesis?* London: Nuffield Provincial Hospitals Trust.

Manton, K.G. and Stallard, E. (1994) Medical demography: interaction of disability dynamics and mortality, in L.G. Martin and S.H. Preston (eds) *Demography of Aging*. Washington, DC: National Academy Press, 217–78.

Munnichs, J.M.A. (1992) Ageing: a kind of autobiography, *European Journal of Gerontology*, 1(4), 244–50.

Phillipson, C. (1991) Inter-generational relations: conflict or consensus in the 21st century?, *Policy and Politics*, 19(1), 27–36.

Shanas, E., Townsend, P., Wedderburn, D., Friis, H., Milhoj, P. and Stehouwer, J. (1965) *Old People in Three Industrial Societies*. London: Routledge & Kegan Paul.

Starr, J.M. (1982) Towards a social phenomenology of aging: studying the self-process in biographical work, *International Journal of Human Development* 16(4), 250–70.

Thompson, P., Itzin, C. and Abendstern, M. (1990) *I Don't Feel Old. The Experience of Later Life*. Oxford: Oxford University Press.

Young, M. and Willmott, P. (1957) *Family and Kinship in East London*. London: Routledge & Kegan Paul.

# 8 GLENDA LAWS

## Spatiality and age relations

*Glenda Laws was an associate professor in the department of geography at Pennsylvania State University. Australian by birth, she had studied and worked in North America for more than ten years, holding positions at the University of Toronto, University of Southern California, and most recently Pennsylvania State. Her work on a variety of social issues – urban poverty, gender, disability, and most recently age – was gaining her an international reputation, and she was viewed by many as one of geography's most able and innovative young academics. Glenda died suddenly on 23 June, 1996, a few days after submitting the final version of the following chapter. She was 37. She was near finishing her book* Social Justice and the State *which will be completed by her husband, Steven Matthews.*

## Introduction

As a point of departure for this chapter, I invite readers to reflect upon an observation by Ralph Waldo Emerson:

> Youth is everywhere in place. Age, like women, requires fit surroundings. Age is comely in coaches, churches, in chambers of State and ceremony, in council chambers, in courts of justice and historical societies . . . But in the rush and uproar of broadway . . . Few envy the consideration enjoyed by the oldest inhabitant. We do not count a man's years until he has nothing else to count . . . In short, the creed of the street is, Old Age is not disgraceful, but immensely disadvantageous.
>
> (Emerson 1862: 135)

This statement suggests that, as we age, our *place* in society, both materially and metaphorically, changes. The material spaces and places in which we live, work and engage in leisure activities are age-graded and, in turn, age is associated with particular places and spaces. Our metaphorical social position also varies with increasing age as old age is peripheralized (its immense disadvantage) into discrete locations, while 'youth is everywhere'. I want to suggest that the seeming simultaneous persistence and transformation of these relationships requires gerontologists to pay greater attention to the reciprocal relations between the social and the spatial if they are to understand the (re)construction of aged identities. My specific objectives in this chapter are (a) to develop the idea of the spatiality of age relations by (b) demonstrating the utility of recent developments in social theory concerning the construction of subjects and identities and (c) examining how aged identities are reflected in and constituted by both materially and discursively constructed built environments. I will argue that identities in general, and aged identities specifically, are fluid and constantly renegotiated. Identities may be imposed on the subject from external sources (e.g. racist, sexist and ageist stereotypes) or they can be self-nominated (acceptance and internalization of these stereotypes) (Hoffmann-Axthelm 1992). Externally defined identities depend upon their being emplaced in some space external to the subject. If self-nomination is involved, then the subject must be embodied or, in Rodaway's (1995: 249) language, located in corporeal places. Subjects and spaces/places, then, are intertwined in a tapestry of relations that produce social identities.

I begin this chapter by describing how social theorists conceptualize the spatial dimensions of identity formation. I then describe several different instances of the intersection of aged identities with particular built environments, in both their material and representational forms. In the conclusion, I will point to other directions that gerontologists interested in the spatiality of aged relations might pursue.

## Spatiality and identity formation

Renewed interest in the spatiality of social life is evident in recent formulations within social theory (Gregory and Urry 1985; Soja 1989; Featherstone and Lash 1995; Pile and Thrift 1995). In reviewing the status of the landscape concept, sociologist Sharon Zukin (1992: 224) summarizes the general thrust of these contributions:

> While landscape's new uses reflect, in part, a widespread awareness of the importance of spatiality (as in 'the landscape of the city'), they also respond to an effort to retrieve spatiality from the domain of geography and analyze it historically, making space the co-equal of time. Space is now considered a dynamic medium that both exerts an influence on history and is shaped by human action. As the confluence of individual biography and structural change, space is potentially an agent that structures society.

To recover the centrality of the spatial in analyses of social change, Ed Soja (1989) develops the concept of the *socio-spatial dialectic*, which describes the links between social processes and the spatial arrangement of society. He calls for a refocusing of social analysis on the reciprocal relations between society and space. Places, like retirement communities or nursing homes, are obviously created by social practices. Over time, people might alter these built environments but, according to Soja's dialectic, we must acknowledge that spaces also alter social practices. For example, once nursing homes were created, attitudes about the appropriate locus of care for certain categories of older people changed. Dear and Wolch (1989) amplify these ideas by describing some of the most common interactions between the social and the spatial. First, the webs of social relations in which we are enmeshed are *constituted* through space. For example, the physical environment might place limits on the type of community that can develop in a particular place and thereby limit potential social interactions. Second, these same social relations are *constrained* by space. Foucault's now well known analysis of the panopticon role of the modern prison illustrates this well. Finally, Dear and Wolch suggest that social relations are *mediated* by space. For example, distances between adult children and their parents make a difference to the frequency and types of interactions in which they can engage.

Spaces are constituted by and constitutive of social relations. Places are defined by Doreen Massey (1994: 5) 'as a particular articulation of those relations, a particular moment in those networks of social relations and understandings.' She goes on to note that the social relations which define a particular place do not operate exclusively in that place. Spatial boundaries are permeable and, within any one location, local and extra-local forces combine to produce the place and its character. Accepting that space is necessarily involved in the constitution of social life and practices raises the question of how it is involved in the creation of the subject. How does the spatial influence identity formation? These concerns have been taken up by researchers in a number of different disciplines, including geography, sociology, women's studies and cultural studies (see Bird *et al.* 1993; Keith and Pile 1993; Featherstone *et al.* 1995; Pile and Thrift 1995). But before addressing the specific question of how identities are spatialized, I will review more general debates about identity formation.

Theorists drawing from Foucault's arguments stress the discursive construction of the subject. Subjects, and the identities they hold or have imposed upon them, whether gendered, racialized or aged, are not ontologically independent of the discourses that describe – and simultaneously construct – them. As the site of subjection, our bodies are coded by cultural discourses. Representations of the body construct the slender, anorectic and nurturing female subject, for example (see Bordo 1993). Similarly, popular and academic discourses construct the racialized body (Omi and Winant 1986). And social gerontologists are increasingly focusing on the implications of discourses about aged bodies for the construction of the aged subject (e.g. Featherstone and Wernick 1995; Laws 1995; Harper in this volume, Chapter 13). However, to focus purely on the symbolic and the representational is limiting. We live and operate in a material world where power relations are institutionalized into social practices. Non-discursive practices, as Foucault realized (see Hennessey 1993), also impact on the creation of the subject. Our identities are structured as much by material acts as they are by discursive practices. The discourses we construct about old age, for example, are often created within material contexts concerned with the 'need' to balance a government budget or to reduce the size of the corporate labour force. In advocating a materialist feminism that is sympathetic to both discursive and non-discursive practices, Rosemary Hennessey (1993: 37) looks for 'a way of thinking about the relationship between language and subjectivity that can explain their connection to other aspects of material life.' Materialist age studies must similarly explain these links and their role in constructing aged subjects. The notion of the spatiality of age relations, with its concern for both material and metaphorical spaces, offers a useful hook on which to hang the beginnings of an appropriate framework.

What roles do space and place play in the fabrication, reconstruction, celebration or repudiation of social identities? In both popular and academic discourses, we often see the association of particular categories of people with particular locations. Identities are spatialized, in that *where* we are says a lot about who we are. There are pervasive links between social and spatial positions; we hold 'geographically specific' stereotypes (Keith and Pile 1993: 3) of people because there are equally powerful stereotypes of places. Elsewhere (Laws 1997) I have argued that there are several dimensions of spatiality – accessibility, mobility, motility, spatial scale and spatial segregation – which are involved in the mutual constitution of places and identities. These need to be only briefly reviewed here:

1 *Accessibility* to particular places, whether a nation state, a residential neighbourhood or a workplace, has impacts for an individual's citizenship status and subsequent identity (e.g. Thomson and Staehli 1997).
2 *Mobility*, both metaphorical and material, between places and social situations is an important marker of one's position relative to others (e.g. Massey 1993).
3 *Motility* refers to an individual body's potential to move (see Young 1989). 'Frail' bodies, whether young or old, impact upon the public identity of people.
4 *Spatial scale* is important (Smith 1993). Our identity in the domestic sphere (a loving grandparent) may be different from that at a national scale (part of the 'greedy geezer' image of older people). When moving between spatial scales, we must be aware of the links between group and individual identities.
5 *Spatial segregation* is produced by limitations on access, mobility and motility and operates on a number of scales. Daphne Spain (1992) notes that spatial segregation of oppressed groups is a key mechanism of social control. As Emerson's quote at the beginning of this chapter illustrates, there are powerful public beliefs about the appropriateness of segregating people of different generations.

Understanding the construction of social and individual identities thus demands that we attend to the spatiality of social life. I now want to illustrate this argument by considering how aged identities are not only the product of particular spatialities but how they also constitute spaces and places.

## Spatialities of old age: examples of residential built environments

The spatiality of age relations is manifested at a number of scales.[1] For the purposes of exposition, I will concentrate on how residential environments construct aged subjects at the same time that the very existence of these environments requires those same subjects. Because retirees, one class of older people, depart from waged labour and its associated built environments, residential environments take on special meaning in the construction of aged subjects. Furthermore, within domestic environments, there has been an increasing separation of generations over the past century. This relatively recent spatial separation of families into different households has reshaped the bonds between grandparents, parents and children, and reconstructed generational differentiations of the body. By choosing different spatial environments at different historical periods, I intend to contribute to a non-essentialist view of old age and focus on the range of aged subjects. I also want to demonstrate the ways in which changing aged identities have resulted in changing spatial environments for older people. Finally, throughout the discussion it is important to keep in mind that there are both material and representational forms of these spatialities, and I will use a particular example to illustrate this point.

### From poorhouse to homes for the aged: redefining old age and its place

My first example illustrates the unstable spatialities of age relations under modernity. Achenbaum (1978) argues that elderly people were generally respected and viewed positively in the United States until the time of the Civil War. Before that time, according to the observers he draws upon, old people were active and productive contributors to US society. After the Civil War, the view of older people changed to a more or less negative one, ageing came to be associated with disease and 'the elderly' were transformed into a perceived burden on society. By the mid-1930s, the view that older people were deserving of social assistance was apparent in the passage of the Social Security Act. The public identity of older people in the USA thus underwent tremendous changes in a relatively short period of time. This transformation in identity was accompanied by a transformation in residential environments for older people, especially those who could not, for whatever reason, live with family. That is, transitions in identity were attended by transitions in spatialities of old age.

Changing attitudes during the second half of the nineteenth century meant that, especially if they were poor, older people were increasingly likely to become residents of large-scaled institutions like poorhouses. Important in this shift was a growing sense that older people were not suitable for the newly industrializing workplace (Achenbaum 1978; also see Laws 1993). In keeping with the comments in the preceding section, being denied access to the new space economy and its waged labour relations had consequences for older people's status as citizens. In the absence of a welfare state, those older people whose families could not, or would not, care for them found their way into the nation's poorhouses (an indicator of downward mobility?), which, over time, and more by default than design, were transformed into homes for the aged.

That poorhouses evolved into homes for the aged had as much to do with discourses about other 'special needs' groups as it did with concerns of older people *per se*. This points to the relational nature of identity and subject formation. Speciality asylums for the mentally ill, the blind and deaf, and other groups grew through the latter part of the nineteenth century in Europe and North America (e.g. Goffman 1961). In addition, the reform movement of the late nineteenth century convincingly argued that children, who had also found their way into the poorhouse system, should be removed to more appropriate environments (i.e. the identity of childhood was associated with the spaces of orphanages rather than the workhouse). The removal of children and other groups left a population of older people in the nation's poorhouses (Achenbaum 1978; Katz 1986). This demographic shift, in conjunction with critics of conditions in the almshouses, presaged the birth of homes for the aged and an explicitly age-segregated element of the North American urban fabric.

Specialized (and spatialized) homes for older people received a real boost from the passage of the Social Security Act, a process that moved the identification of aged subjects away from the local scale into the political realm of the nation state. Older people had found their way to the poorhouse because of their poverty. At the turn of the century, advocates argued that the increasingly affluent industrial society should provide a pension system for people forced to retire from the manufacturing-based economy. Increasingly a new identity of the *deserving* aged was being publicly defined, and it was explicitly *not* associated with the poorhouse environment. John Lapp (1925: 28) argued that 'It will stand for a long time as a blot upon our history that no better outlook has been afforded for the worthy aged than the associations provided in the county almshouse. The old age pension system . . . will take out of the almshouse the worthy aged and it will provide for thousands who now live in an uncertain and unhappy existence outside.' The implementation of the Social Security Act signalled that, within the nation state, older people were deemed worthy of public support, regardless of how they might be conceived within particular localities or households.

The Social Security Act provided a firm financial foundation for proprietary homes by guaranteeing an income for older people. Achenbaum (1978: 151) succinctly summarizes one set of outcomes:

> The authors of the act, who by and large, rejected the almshouse method of providing for aged dependents, drafted and successfully defended a provision denying direct assistance to poor house inmates. A hitherto unnoticed institution, the 'rest home', benefited from the situation because it could offer a residence and care for old people on public assistance without contravening Title I [of the Social Security Act]. Many former (or potential) poor farm residents thus relocated in proprietary homes.

Indeed, since the passage of the Social Security Act, and especially since the implementation of Medicare, there has been an explosion in the number of residential facilities for older people. The financial security of many of these depends upon federal government support. Property owners in 'the land of old age' (Laws 1993) are keenly watching debates in the US Congress about how to deal with a growing deficit. Their futures are closely tied to the future of programmes directed at older Americans.

Between the Civil War and 1935, changes in discursive constructions of older people were matched by changes in the material spaces in which they participated. The view that they were not suited to the harsh demands of the industrial economy removed them from the workplace and relegated them to residential spaces. For the poorest, especially those deemed less than worthy, these spaces were not intimate domestic spaces of a family home but were rather institutional spaces of the poorhouse, designed initially with a different clientele in mind. As discourses about other occupants of the poorhouse changed, these institutions increasingly became built environments for old people, and thus were able to maintain their position in the urban built environment for a little longer.[2] Finally, with the construction of a class of worthy old people, more 'respectable' spaces[3] created by both proprietary and non-profit organizations evolved to house the newly identified recipients of social security, an indication of their (or their spouses') ties to the labour market and thus evidence of their respectability and status as citizens.

### Sun City and the discursive construction of aged subjects

In contrast to this historically distant example of changing discourses during modernity, my second example will focus on the discursive construction of aged identities in representations of Sun City retirement communities – exemplary of 'designer' retirement landscapes under postmodernity (Holdsworth and Laws 1994). That is, in this particular example, I will not say anything about the material form of the landscape but focus instead on its discursive construction and how this in turn constructs aged identities (this discussion is developed more fully in Laws 1995).

To be successful, Sun City communities depend on a particular identity and, to ensure their success, they must actively construct this identity. One of the most powerful tools for doing this is the marketing of Sun Cities through a variety of print and video media as well as sites on the World Wide Web. These sources represent the material place as well as the identities and bodies whom the developers seek as residents. Thus, identities are spatialized and places become embodied in marketing representations. Whereas in the preceding example I focused on particular residence types (the poorhouse, the home for the aged), in this case I want to move outward in terms of spatial scale and think about the construction of a community and the identities associated with it. The Sun City advertising literature is very much geared to selling the community as much as any one particular house design. It constructs bodies whose motility and carriage will 'fit' the community's image.

As with most real estate advertising, the image of Sun City is a place populated by active and happy people. Sun City is a landscape to be consumed. Typically, consumption is represented as taking place (and consumption does indeed take place) around swimming, golf or some other social activity. This place requires and constructs a particular type of body and subject – one that is ready, willing and able to be busy while relaxing. Coloured brochures show golfing couples on a fairway in front of an artificial pond (complete with an artificial waterfall). The palm trees and mountains are in the background both actually and metaphorically; they appear incidental to the golfing needs of potential residents. Other images include a team of women synchronized swimmers, lawn bowlers and a couple in formal wear enjoying 'fun-filled evenings out on the town in neighboring Palm Springs'. Modes of motility and comportment popularly (though by no means necessarily) associated with youth are central to the representation of Sun City.[4] The level of activity in these images suggests that the reader could be perusing a brochure for a resort instead of a retirement community. The resort image is continued in an advertisement for 'a very affordable resort-style getaway' that invites potential residents to 'try it before you buy it'. Packages 'include deluxe accommodations, free 18 holes of golf, and access to our multi-million dollar recreational facilities, where you can play tennis, lounge by the pools, and more.' Like cruise ships, Sun Cities are relatively self-contained. But as with a cruise, residents can 'go ashore' to purchase goods and services not available on board.

Location is of critical importance if these excursions are to be viable. Sun Cities tend to be located on the outskirts of mid-sized urban centres. Residents thereby have access to a range of the lifestyle trappings necessary for consumption. Accessibility to nearby resources is announced in brochures which reassure potential residents that their new communities will not result in social isolation. Shopping centres, health facilities and restaurants are all within a short drive. Sun City communities are spatially segregated from the problems of big city life, but never so far away that the residents cannot take advantage of urban amenities. Location is important not so much because of surrounding 'natural' environments but because it allows ready participation in those consumptive practices, 'in which life and the consumer accoutrements which make it possible are constantly stylised and re-stylised to achieve a pleasant effect' (Featherstone and Hepworth 1990: 374).

In the promotional representations emphasis is placed on the notion of community. Sun Cities are, for example, represented as playing an influential role in the surrounding area. In one brochure, the chairman and chief executive officer of the Del Webb Corporation describes Sun Cities as projects 'which enhance the lifestyle of neighboring communities and exist in harmony with the local environment.' Another brochure boasts, 'Community pride runs strong here, too – you couldn't ask for people to take better care of their neighborhoods.' The conflation of people, pride and place is an important component to a sense of community. Several of the Palm Springs brochures open with the comment that 'Del Webb wants the residents of Sun City Palm Springs to be informed about their community.' The advertising brochures-cum-newsletters provide residents (present and future) with details of, for example, the fragile environment of the Coachella Valley in which Sun City Palm Springs is located.

The representations of the Sun City community are thus geared to a very particular embodied identity – an active, affluent, senior population. But such identities were not simply waiting for some group like the Del Webb Corporation to build them a community or two. This identity has been actively constructed over the past two decades as business interests recognized the windfall available to them through the private pensions and social security benefits negotiated during the post-war economic boom. The Del Webb Corporation and many other businesses have worked hard to construct a discursive identity that people would adopt in their material lives. Real estate developers have been particularly cognizant of the need to spatialize these identities in order to make their own projects profitable. As these identities are constructed and adopted by an increasing number of people, demand for lifestyle retirement communities also increases.[5]

## Space, identities and the transformation of old age

My purpose in this chapter has been to draw attention to the spatiality of age relations. This is not to say simply that old people live in space. There is a much more powerful role for the spatial in the creation of aged identities. The experience of being old, for example, varies according to one's environment. Situation can thus actively affect ageing. That age relations are constituted in, mediated by and constrained by space begs a refocusing of attention in social gerontology. Ralph Waldo Emerson's observations from more than a century ago highlight the importance of focusing on the spatial constitution of age relations. I have built on this point by stressing the mutual constitution of place and age relations.

Clearly there are important links between built environments, representations of lifestyles and stages of the life course, and the construction of aged identities. Changing constructions of old age as well as actual improvements in health and longevity have challenged the arbitrariness of chronological age divisions in popular representations of 'young' and 'old'. Age-segregated environments are integral to the process of identity formation by both older individuals (who might accept the identity of an active retiree) and other social groups who perceive elderly people in particular ways. Multiple spatialities and social practices define age relations and these have changed since Emerson penned his observation. Consider changes in the relations between age and worksites. On the one hand, the abolition of mandatory retirement means that older people will not necessarily vacate the workplace in the future. On the other hand, early retirement programmes further complicate the picture – 'retirees' are now chronologically younger and are encouraged to be involved in activities once thought the exclusive domain of younger people. Workplace day-care centres and senior volunteers in schools represent challenges to whom we expect to see in particular places.

One interesting point that emerges from the evolution of new built environments for older people is the fact that age is used to sell certain commodities. Retirement communities are an example of product differentiation. At one level, they amount to little more than one form of real estate development. But by segmenting the real estate market, these communities imbue ageing and retirement with new, and to some extent positive, meanings. So, although Mike Featherstone (1995: 230) is correct to note 'the disempowerment which follows from a reduction of the symbolic capital of the body with the onset of old age', we must be cautious of seeing this reduction occurring in all aspects of aged identities. New landscapes have been created to house ageing bodies, and these landscapes are clearly profitable. They are an important part of the construction of what Moody (1993: xx) has referred to as a postmodern lifecourse, one that is as much concerned with consumption as it is with production. While Moody draws attention to the consumption regimes that surround the postmodern life course, future research must also consider the role of new, 'postmodern' technologies which allow, to a certain degree, 'disembodied' experiences in '"nonplace" worlds [of] . . . simulated environments' (Featherstone 1995: 233). What are the implications of the virtual world for the lived experience of the life course and the spatiality of age relations? Will space and place become less important in the construction of aged identities? What are the consequences for those people who do not have access to these new 'nonplace worlds'? Cyberspace is not readily available to the poor in either the developed or developing nations of the world.

A remaining task is to consider the ideological work being done by the landscapes of old age. Old age is a contested category (Laws 1994) and residential environments that serve older people are part of ongoing contests and negotiations. Just as the poorhouse represented a particular iteration of late nineteenth-century moral codes, so the designer retirement community sends out messages not only about 'successful' retirement but also about wise investment strategies while one is part of the labour force. Planned retirement communities have grown in tandem with the multitude of pre-retirement financial planning services that are now part of consumer culture in the United States. Working-age people are bombarded with information about the importance of planning early for future retirement. Being able to make choices about one's housing situation in the future depends to a large part on discipline and personal responsibility while working. The vast majority of older people do not find their way into either the designer communities produced by large property developers or the late twentieth-century version of housing for low-income older people. The majority stay in their own homes. Home ownership as a form of financial security in one's old age is also part of a powerful ideology about personal responsibility which has been one of the main forces structuring the spatiality of North American cities. Growing old in the family home is thus as important to the construction of aged identities as is growing old in a poorhouse or a retirement community. Different spatial environments provide one mechanism for the differentiation of aged identities, at least those aspects of identity that are defined in terms of consumption and residential segregation. However, in closing, we must of course note that not all groups of older people have the resources that allow them to choose which of the identities they wish to wear. Future research should attend to the links between social power, prestige and the restructuring of the land of old age.

## Notes

1  For example, elder abuse is indicative of power relations operating within a household, although structured by broader forces. Programmes operated by sub-national

governments might direct more or less funds to young or old people. Similarly, at the national scale, policies are very important in the constructing of aged identities. Cultural practices which dominate nation states are also important. In many Asian nations, for example, older people remain within the households of extended families.

2  While the institution of the nineteenth century is largely a relic, it is worth noting that criticism of some nursing homes suggest some may still convey an institutional setting – if not in architectural detail then in treatment of residents within the walls.

3  Many contemporary observers praised private-sector initiatives. Private homes were 'far superior to the public almshouses [since the] heads of these homes are not only superior to the almshouse stewards, but the institutional matron or superintendent generally tries to make the place a real home' (Epstein 1938: 514). *The New York Times* noted that 'happily, with the foundation of private homes for the aged, thousands have been spared this doom [of entering the almshouse]'.

4  It is important at this point to remind ourselves that essentialist images of either youth or old age are socially constructed. There is no intrinsic reason why older people should not be fit and active and indeed most are. However, I am interested in the juxtaposition of stereotypical representations.

5  Recognition that the affluent active retiree's body may deteriorate biologically to the point of his or her being identified as a 'frail elderly' individual has resulted in the creation of another new residential environment for older people: campus-style retirement communities that provide both independent living and nursing home environments (Laws 1993).

## References

Achenbaum, W.A. (1978) *Old Age in the New Land*. Boulder, CO: Westview Press.

Bird, J., Curtis, B., Putnam, T., Robertson, G. and Tickner, L. (eds) (1993) *Mapping the Futures: Local Cultures, Global Change*. London: Routledge.

Bordo, S. (1993) *Unbearable Weight: Feminism, Western Culture and the Body*. Berkeley: University of California Press.

Dear, M. and Wolch, J. (1989) How territory shapes social life, in J. Wolch, J. and M. Dear (eds) *The Power of Geography: How Territory Shapes Social Life*. Boston: Unwin Hyman.

Emerson, R.W. (1862) Old age, *Atlantic Monthly*, 9, 134–8.

Epstein, A. (1938) *Insecurity: a Challenge of America*. New York: Random House.

Featherstone, M. (1995) Post-bodies, aging and virtual reality, in M. Featherstone, M. and A. Wernick (eds) *Images of Aging: Cultural Representations of Later Life*. London: Routledge.

Featherstone, M. and Hepworth, M. (1990) The mask of ageing and the postmodern life course, in M. Featherstone, M. Hepworth and B. Turner (eds) *The Body: Social Process and Cultural Theory*. London: Sage.

Featherstone, M. and Lash, S. (1995) Globalisation, modernity and the spatialisation of social theory: an introduction, in M. Featherstone, S. Lash and R. Robertson (eds) *Global Modernities*. London: Sage Publications.

Featherstone, M., Lash, S. and Robertson, R. (eds) (1995) *Global Modernities*. London: Sage Publications.

Featherstone, M. and Wernick, A. (eds) 1995 *Images of Aging: Cultural Representations of Later Life*. London: Routledge.

Goffman, E. (1961) *Asylums: Essays on the Social Situation of Mental Patients*. Harmondsworth: Penguin.

Gregory, D. and Urry, J. (eds) (1985) *Social Relations and Spatial Structures*. London: Macmillan.

Hennessey, R. (1993) *Material Feminism and the Politics of Discourse*. New York: Routledge.

Hoffmann-Axthelm, D. (1992) Identity and reality: the end of the philosophical immigration officer, in S. Lash and J. Friedman (eds) *Modernity and Identity*. Oxford: Blackwell.

Holdsworth, D. and Laws, G. (1994) Landscapes of old age in coastal British Columbia, *Canadian Geographer*, 38(2), 162–9.

Katz, M. (1986) *In the Shadow of the Poorhouse: a Social History of Welfare in America*. New York: Basic Books.

Keith, M. and Pile, S. (1993) Introduction Part 1: The politics of place, in M. Keith and S. Pile (eds) *Place and the Politics of Identity*. London: Routledge.

Lapp, J.A. (1925) Growing insistence upon pensions instead of institutional care for aged dependents, *American Labor Legislation Review*, 15, 23–9.

Laws, G. (1993) 'The land of old age': society's changing attitudes toward urban built environments for elderly people, *Annals, Association of American Geographers*, 83(4), 672–93.

Laws, G. (1994) Contested meanings, the built environment and aging in place, *Environment and Planning A*, 26, 1787–802.

Laws, G. (1995) Embodiment and emplacement: identities, representation and landscape in Sun City retirement communities, *International Journal of Aging and Human Development*, 40(4), 253–80.

Laws, G. (1997) Women's life courses, spatial mobility and state policies, in S. Roberts, H. Nast, H. and J.P. Jones (eds) *Thresholds in Feminist Geography*. Savage, MD: Rowman and Littlefield.

Massey, D. (1993) Power-geometry and a progressive sense of space, in J. Bird, B. Curtis, T. Putnam, G. Robertson and L. Tickner (eds) *Mapping the Futures: Local Cultures, Global Change*. London: Routledge.

Massey, D. (1994) *Space, Place, Gender*. Minneapolis: University of Minnesota Press.

Moody, H. (1993) Overview: what is critical gerontology and why is it important, in T.R. Cole, W.A. Achenbaum, P. Jakobi and R. Kastenbaum (eds) *Voices and Visions of Aging. Toward a Critical Gerontology*. New York: Springer.

Omi, M. and Winant, H. (1986) *Racial Formation in the United States*. New York: Routledge.

Pile, S. and Thrift, N. (eds) (1995) *Mapping the Subject: Geographies of Cultural Transformation*. London: Routledge.

Rodaway, P. (1995) Exploring the subject in hyper-reality, in S. Pile, and N. Thrift, (eds) *Mapping the Subject: Geographies of Cultural Transformation*. London: Routledge.

Smith, N. (1993) Homeless/global: scaling places, in J. Bird, B. Curtis, T. Putnam, G. Robertson and L. Tickner (eds) *Mapping the Futures: Local Cultures, Global Change*. London: Routledge.

Soja, E. (1989) *Postmodern Geographies*. London: Verso.

Spain, D. (1992) *Gendered Spaces*. Chapel Hill, NC: University of North Carolina Press.

Thomson, A. and Staehli, L. (forthcoming) Citizenship, community, and struggles for public space, *The Professional Geographer*.

Young, I.M. (1989) Throwing like a girl: a phenomenology of feminine body comportment, motility, and spatiality, in J. Allen and I.M. Young (eds) *The Thinking Muse: Feminism and Modern French Philosophy*. Bloomington: Indiana University Press.

Young, I.M. (1990) *Justice and the Politics of Difference*. Princeton, NJ: Princeton University Press.

Zukin, S. (1992) *Landscapes of Power: from Detroit to Disney World*. Berkeley: University of California Press.

ANDREW BLAIKIE AND MIKE HEPWORTH

# Representations of old age in painting and photography

The more we know about literature and history, the more we can master the significance of visual work. The greater our knowledge of a period, the easier it is to penetrate the spirit of its artistic texts. But we must have no illusions: many of its essential meanings escape us. A vast number of these meanings, with their cultural, social, allegorical and symbolic stratifications are lost once and for all. Because of this we may be tempted to fall back on a false interpretation, a surrogate which consists of a reading based, not on the work of art itself, but on what we would like it to be.

(Zeri 1990)

## Introduction

This chapter is divided into two sections. The first examines images of old age in Victorian paintings (selected from the period 1837–1901) and the second examines images of old age in twentieth-century photography, in particular from the period 1950 to the present day. Drawing on examples from these two sources, we argue for a social constructionist analysis of visual images of old age. Our core argument is that visual images are not simply direct copies, made with varying degrees of skill and accuracy, from an independently observed external reality, but are, as the word 'image' suggests, the combined product of technical skill and the human imagination. The technical ability to create visual images works in the service of imagined ideas and beliefs which determine both the direction of the painter's or photographer's interest and the subsequent interpretations which may be made by the wider public of the resulting image. If the workings of the human imagination are motivated and shaped by culturally determined ideas and practices, then the range of visual images produced during any particular historical period provides us with important information concerning the ways in which visual perceptions of the external appearance of old age (as represented, for example, in a portrait of Queen Victoria in later life or a photograph of an older couple in a country cottage) are constructed. Images of old age are not therefore timeless reflections of some essential reality of old age, whose meaning is fixed once and for all, but are culturally determined representations of the beliefs of the time concerning the nature of the ageing process and the role of older people in society. Equally significantly, they are also evidence of key ideas about the social functions of visual images and their role in public life. At the same time, as the introductory quotation above indicates, when we attempt to make any kind of reading of visual images of old age, especially those constructed in periods other than our own, we must be keenly aware that we are reading these images through the lens of present-day assumptions, ideals and values concerning the process of growing older in the late twentieth century. We must always bear in mind that visual images are never 'innocent' but, in an archaeological sense, comprise several layers of interpretation and reinterpretation; as such, they constitute the social imagination of old age.

## Victorian culture and the 'drama of modernity'

There are two main reasons why Victorian culture offers a particularly interesting case study of the social imagination of old age. The first is the key role played in nineteenth-century society by 'the drama of modernization' (Eisenman 1994: 7). One significant aspect of this drama is an acceleration of processes of scientific and technological innovation and the application of scientific thinking to human life. In the biological sciences, Darwin's painstakingly researched theory of the origins of the species, itself the product of a strand of nineteenth-century evolutionary thought, argued for incontrovertible evidence that human beings were not the special creation of God and that life was essentially an endless struggle for the survival of the fittest. The vision of the natural world as a benign homeland for the superior human race was destabilized by geologists who no longer saw evidence in rock formations of permanence and timelessness, but rather signs of massive upheaval, discontinuity and flux. In this complex cultural climate a congruence emerged between concepts of biological life as a battlefield and social life, especially economic life, as a competitive struggle. To survive this struggle, to display moral worth, the individual had to demonstrate physical fitness and prowess. Reliance on the survival power of the human body inevitably produced a climate of increasing anxiety about the physical wear and tear of old age, and it is no coincidence that during this period concerted efforts were made to apply the principles of modern science to the ageing process in the hope of discovering the underlying biological causes of ageing.

One problem was that developments in the scientific analysis of human life did not completely displace more traditional religious perspectives, with the result that the tension created between these two modes of conceptualizing the meaning and purpose of human life generated considerable social and personal anxiety. The common response to this state of cultural stress was to attempt to get the best of both possible worlds by celebrating the practical achievements of science and technology, while simultaneously preserving the sacred and mysterious. If science and economics had produced empirically verifiable evidence of life as a materialistic battle for the 'survival of the fittest', it was still possible to 'create intense little havens' for the cultivation of a comfortable spiritual security (Bartram 1985: 39). As we shall see below, these tensions between science and sentiment are particularly evident in one strand of Victorian painting, where a prominent image of old age is a nostalgic vision of growing old gracefully in a comforting rural haven far removed from the harsh realities of struggling for an existence in the limbo of the heavily industrialized big city: a moralistic vision fittingly described as 'rural nostalgia' (Morrison 1989).

The second reason for our choice of the Victorian period is also related to the 'drama of modernity'. One of the central characteristics of modernization during the nineteenth century was the increasingly significant role of visual imagery in social life. It was during this period that technical advances in the ability to reproduce and circulate visual images on a massive scale produced what has been described as a '"media explosion" – the proliferation of mass-produced, printed images (first lithographs, later photographs) pioneered in France but spread throughout Europe, England, and America' (Williams 1995: 3). As the sheer number of visual images in circulation multiplied, so the 'habit of visualisation' (Sillars 1995: 3) was cultivated and the public became progressively skilled in interpreting the meanings of pictures in terms of the dynamic interaction between pictures and words.

Aspects of this increasingly complex and 'layered' process of visual sensitization can be detected in the unprecedented public interest in painting which became evident during the mid-Victorian period. A significant characteristic of nineteenth-century painting is the expanding popular appeal of art galleries and exhibitions. Victorian intellectuals were not slow to appreciate the educative role of contemporary painting. Art galleries, which attracted huge crowds of viewers, were explicitly opened to the general public as a force for moral education and the recognition of art as a process of communication between patron, public and artist fostered a condition of mutual interdependence. Under the tutelage of art critics, the 'observer spectator' emerged, skilled in interpreting the significance of the contents of a particular painting. Objects in a room, furnishings, clothing and the human characters were all scrutinized in order to assess their social and, above all, their moral qualities (Cowling 1989). Towards the end of the century, entrepreneurs such as Lord Lever, the inventor of Sunlight Soap and a prominent patron of art, adapted paintings of the day to his advertising campaigns and recruited popular artists who were willing to produce illustrations for his soap advertisements. One notable feature of his patronage is the use of images of older women – a variation of the 'granny' figure – to popularize the use of washday soap among the lower classes (Hepworth 1995a). Typically this figure, expressly constructed to cultivate an enthusiasm for soap among the lower classes, is an energetic old woman, enthusiastically attacking a mound of washing and not infrequently surrounded by a collection of lively children. Above all, this image of a working-class woman does not display old age as disengagement from women's work but actively celebrates prolonged active life.

The popular interest in the role of painting in cultivating the moral imagination is indicated by the extensive patronage of Queen Victoria, whose private collection includes a number of paintings in which old age is a central theme. Among her collection of family portraits and those of public servants and faithful retainers, for example, is at least one which she specifically commissioned because the subject, Augusta, Duchess of Cambridge, painted by Heinrich von Angeli, was growing older and the Queen wished to preserve her image. Typically for the period, the Duchess is dressed as a widow: a black dress and cap with a white lace fringe and scarf. The artist reported that he experienced some difficulty in carrying out the work because it was 'so dark, and she so suffering and ailing, and so much movement about' (Millar 1992: 7). Looking back on this portrait, and reading it in the light of the comment of the time, it is not difficult to detect the signs of suffering patiently endured and to share Queen Victoria's perception of this painting as an icon of virtuous old age.

Other less personal paintings in Queen Victoria's collection also reflect the characteristically Victorian interpretation of the virtues of old age (what we now tend to describe as 'positive ageing' (Hepworth 1995b). These include Andrew MacCallum's *The Upward Path of Life* (1883) (Millar 1992), a Victorian version of the image of life as a series of 'ages' or 'stages', the origins of which can be traced back to classical antiquity. This painting comprises three canvasses in a single frame, neatly dividing life into three stages: 'Youth, Morning', 'Manhood, Midday' and 'Old Age, Evening'. The painting is essentially allegorical: all the human figures are very small and completely subordinate to the landscape, which itself is secondary to a specific moral function. The third painting, 'Old Age, Evening', displays that traditional symbol of old age, an old man with a stick, making his way in the twilight towards a church. Unlike the portrait of the Duchess of Cambridge, designed to celebrate the particular virtues of an identified member of the royal court circle, he is indistinguishable as an individual.

## Old age in Victorian painting

Our brief examination of specific images of old age in Queen Victoria's private collection provides some evidence of the strong moralistic strand in Victorian painting, a strand with close links to the broader tradition of religious thought which continued, as we have noted, to persist throughout the period in dramatic tension with scientific and pragmatic attitudes. Such tension is one indication of the complexity of Victorian culture which can no longer be conceptualized as a unitary structure. The upsurge of critical interest in Victorian art over the past few decades has made scholars much more aware of the competing movements and modes of expression in Victorian art and the complex social tensions which this art reflects. Put simply, there is not one school of Victorian painting but several. This means that the quest for images of old age and the messages they convey to gerontologists must be carried out with extreme care. In particular, it is necessary for us to be on our guard against glib overgeneralization. Research into the social construction of images of ageing and old age reveals that it is dangerously misleading to draw upon paintings and photographs as a resource for an understanding of the nature of the ageing process without detailed analysis of the historical cultures within which paintings are produced and the motives, expectations and perspectives of the people concerned (Featherstone and Wernick 1995; Hepworth 1995c; Featherstone and Hepworth 1996). At the same time, it is possible to detect certain significant themes or 'framings' of representations of later life in Victorian painting: themes which continue to exert a powerful influence on the social imagination and to influence perceptions and experiences of ageing up to the present day. Many of the images of old age which are prominent in the repertoire of visual images we draw upon in contemporary society to give meaning to later life can be traced back to the Victorian period. The aim of this section of the chapter, therefore, is to outline in terms of framing practices at least some of these complexities and thus to highlight some of the broader social processes at work in the social construction of images of old age.

*Framing old age*

Paintings are ways of 'framing' perceptions. The process involves, first, the selection of a specific visual field and, second, establishing boundaries around that field. Frames are techniques for giving shape to a visual image, and as such they 'serve to exhibit and display' (Kay and Rubin 1994: 3). The practice of framing old age within a painting does not therefore simply consist of enclosing a filled surface (canvas, paper etc.) within the boundaries of a picture frame and then hanging the framed picture in a selected site (itself a significant social process: Pointon 1993), but also refers to the form taken by the visualization of old age within specifically created or imagined settings which are realizations of the artist's imagination. In this sense, framing includes not only the repertoire of symbols employed by the artist but also the preferred context and mode of artistic expression. A very good example here is Whistler's world famous painting of his mother. Since its first exhibition in 1872, this painting has come to occupy a prominent place in the popular imagination and continues to be referred to as a positive symbol of graceful feminine old age, more specifically a 'maternal archetype' (Bendiner 1985: 80). Yet Whistler's choice of title for the painting, *Arrangement in Grey and Black No. 1: The Artist's Mother*, suggests something completely different. In the artist's perception, as the number indicates, this painting is only the first of a series of shapes and colours, a creative 'arrangement' rather than a 'realistic' representation of later life. In the words of Julian Treuherz (1993: 138), although Whistler 'was returning to nature for inspiration, he stressed artifice rather than realism or personal feeling, employing deliberately restricted, sometimes almost monochromatic colour schemes and simplified shapes, aiming to capture the essence but not the details of a scene.' Such was Whistler's concern with the values of aestheticism that he designed his own picture frames and went to considerable lengths to hang his paintings in what he regarded as appropriate settings (Treuherz 1993).

These provisional observations offer a brief glimpse of the range of artistic styles in evidence throughout the Victorian period. Within this diversity of constructions, old age is richly represented and we give below *six* variations in the framing of old age in Victorian painting. Similar categories may be applied to Victorian photographs (see Blaikie 1994). The themes are as follows:

1 Paintings, such as the previously cited portrait of the Duchess of Cambridge, where older people are the focus of interest *because* they have lived a long time. As we have already noted, such paintings were usually framed in order to demonstrate the physiognomic evidence of a virtuous character. In this reading, the representation of the wrinkles of old age fixes and enhances virtue, just as it can in the opposite case expose crime and vice (Hepworth 1995d).

Another quite different example, in this case in the form of narrative painting, is Frank Bramley's *After Fifty Years* (1893). A meal has been served outside in honour of the Golden Wedding of an old couple, who occupy the left foreground. Side by side, they are the focus of attention of the guests: 'People are beginning to rise from the table to watch two shy young children, presumably grandchildren, or perhaps even great grandchildren, as they hesitate in the act of presenting bouquets to the old lady' (Fox and Greenacre 1979: 64). With clear connections with the Darby and Joan theme of idyllic married old age, the sentiments stimulated by this form of painting were widely respected and, indeed, expected by viewers.

2 'Ages of life' paintings in which old age is not the central concern, but the natural ending to the biblical 'three score years and ten'. The most obvious of these is *The Seven Ages of Man*, as, for example, painted by Mulready during 1835–8. Reference has already been made to the allegorical function of Andrew MacCallum's *The Upward Path of Life*; in Mulready's version there can be found a pictorial representation of Shakespeare's 'seven ages of man' speech in *As You Like It*, where his character, Jacques, famously spells out the key stages of the life course of a typical man. During the Victorian period other artists, such as Ford Maddox Brown and the Pre-Raphaelites, produced versions (Pointon 1986), and it is important to remember that complementary versions of the 'seven ages of woman' were also produced, reflecting, not surprisingly, conventional beliefs concerning the woman's place in the home.

One of the most appropriate places for old people to be in Victorian painting is in the home, and similar life course themes to that of the 'ages of man' can be found in paintings of family scenes, where older people are an integral feature although they do not occupy centre stage. In their study of images of childhood in British art, Holdsworth and Crossley (1992) comment on the peripheral position occupied by the grandfather in W.P. Frith's *Many Happy Returns of the Day* (1856). In this birthday celebration of a comfortable middle-class family, the grandfather is moved away from the main action at the dining table into an armchair at the side, although the grandmother is seated at the table with a child at either side. This positioning, the authors suggest, 'may suggest that the artist wishes to comment upon the continuity and renewal of the family – the young coming up and replacing the mature, who may then rest in old age' (Holdsworth and Crossley 1992: 100).

3 Paintings in which old age or the life course is not the central concern but older people are included in order to complement, as in (2), a broader theme or to emphasize a moral message. A good example is H.H. La Thangue's *The Man with the Scythe* (1896). In this painting the centre of interest is a little girl supported by pillows in a chair outside a cottage. A woman, presumably the mother, is leaning in concern towards the little girl who has died. In the background is the figure of an old farm worker walking past the gate, a scythe over his shoulder. Here, as Linda Nochlin (1990: 86) has observed, 'the symbolic meaningfulness appropriate to death imagery may be included in the world of everyday actuality by presenting it as mere coincidence . . . within the setting of a contemporary lower-class garden a mother . . . leans over the chair of her little girl who has just stopped breathing . . . while at the same moment, viewed in the background of the picture, an old man comes by.' La Thangue belonged to the naturalist school of rural painting, and his play on an everyday image of agriculture labour and the traditional symbolism of death made a powerful impact.

4 Paintings explicitly depicting a variety of human 'types' in everyday life, and which include, without any explicit allegorical intent, older men and women as a commonplace feature of the social scene. The most obvious examples are found in the work of W.P. Frith, whose panoramic views of Victorian life, which included *Life at the Seaside: Ramsgate Sands* (1854) and *The Derby Day* (1856–8), proved so popular with the Victorian public. It is interesting to note that exact reproductions of the physiognomic lineaments of old age were generally regarded as a purely technical challenge by Victorian artists. In his *Autobiography and Reminiscences* (New York, two volumes, 1888), Frith recorded his preoccupation with the technical difficulties of painting the physiognomy of old age and, commenting on the visual content of *Ramsgate Sands*, the art historian Mary Cowling (1989: 225) has observed that 'the old women throughout the painting . . . are particularly well conceived.' In such paintings older people blend into the social scene, and are, in this sense at least, simply a part of the overall visual scene, although old age does have its part to play: in this instance of constructing a 'natural' or conventional reading of the nature of human life.

5 Scenes in which older people exemplify a specific role for those in later life, or one which older people can continue to play when past their youth. Examples of the former include the comforting role of the older widow when her young daughter or daughter-in-law has lost her husband in an accident. The Victorian favourite was undoubtedly an accident at sea, and there are numerous versions of this theme, several of which were painted, like H.H. La Thangue's paintings of rural life, from direct observation of the hazardous lives of poor people. Frank Bramley's *A Hopeless Dawn* (1888) made him famous, and is described by Raymond Lister (1966: 140) as follows: 'The younger woman is on the point of collapse, and the older woman cradles her tenderly, for she has known, from long and bitter experience, the recurrence of this tragedy.'

Examples of the continuation of working roles into later life include John P. Burr's *The Village Barber* (1881), which shows an old man with spectacles and a white chin beard cutting the hair of a young boy in a rustic barber's shop.

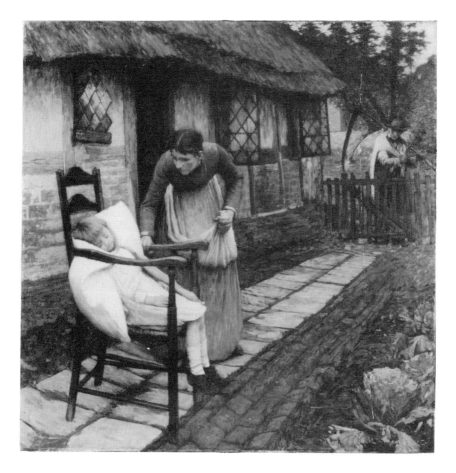

H. H. La Thangue, 'The man with the scythe', 1896. Reproduced with the permission of the Tate Gallery, London.

6 Paintings which draw upon old age during the course of an expression of aesthetic value, which may include efforts to overcome a technical problem. We have referred above to Frith's interest in the technical problems surrounding the portrayal of old age and to Whistler's development of a new style of painting which challenged existing conventions. Artistic challenges to conventional ways of imaging old age have an important part to play in constructing new images of ageing and are explicitly evident in the late twentieth century.

## Painting and photography

Victoria's ascendancy to the throne in 1837 coincided almost exactly with the invention of photography. The new medium provoked an intense debate about the relationship between painting and modern technology, which reflected in part the pervasive tension between religion and science in Victorian culture. The tension in this instance was one between science and art: Science – photography – as the ability to capture the essence of reality, and art as a creative perceptual response to the natural world and to experience. On one level a close symbiotic relationship developed between art and science. Examples can be found in such photographs of old age as Henry Peach Robinson's *Day's Work Done* (1877), which in content and construction closely resembles a genre painting. This is a cottage scene with resonances of Darby and Joan. An old rustic couple of the kind we encountered in some of the paintings we discussed above are portrayed surrounded by the paraphernalia of the self-sufficient life: gardening implements, baskets of vegetables, buckets, fishing tackle and potted plants in the window. He is reading the Bible, his finger painstakingly tracing the words, and she has paused attentively from her sewing to catch the sacred words.

Another picture by the same photographer, which proved extremely popular when exhibited, is *Fading Away* (1858). This one is less focused on old age as such but, as a death bed scene, is a reflection on the theme of the closeness of old age to death. On this particular death bed is a young girl surrounded by her loved ones, including an old lady, presumably her grandmother, whose gaze is fixed intently on the dying girl's face. The association of old age with death, in this instance intended as a source of comfort, is also, of course, a reflection of the reality of death during the nineteenth century, when infant mortality was high and old age was still closely associated, albeit with increasing ambivalence, with spirituality by virtue of advancing years to heaven. Although quite different in content, the theme of this photograph is similar to that of Frederick Walker's painting *The Harbour of Refuge* (1872). Here an old and stooping woman, leaning on the arm of a young woman, walks slowly through the garden of a rural almshouse. The inclusion of an everyday image of a man with a scythe who is mowing the lawn once again represents death.

## Old age and contemporary photography

How far can our analysis be applied to the imagery of old age in the visual arts today? As an example, we now turn to contemporary photography (1950–96). Over the past 150 years, technical innovations have revolutionized the production and circulation of visual images. John Berger has noted that 'In the age of pictorial reproduction the meaning of paintings is no longer attached to them; their meaning becomes transmittable: that is to say it becomes information of a sort, and, like all information, is either put to use or ignored' (Berger 1972: 24). Not only this, but the advent of photography has produced new sorts of information, images capable of manipulation in an infinite variety of ways. Bolton adds: 'the photograph is polysemic . . . it has no single independent meaning, but many possible meanings depending upon context and use . . . [but] just as a social context makes certain readings possible, it can make other readings *im*possible. Institutions authorize certain meanings and dismiss, even silence, others. Thus there is a politics of interpretation that one contends with immediately, whether one knows it or not. To interpret a photograph, or any cultural object, is to negotiate a sea of choices already made' (Bolton 1992: 281). The implications for the understanding of ageing are clear, yet surprisingly little cognizance has been taken of such observations: images of old age tend to be accepted as true likenesses, testimony to the wholly unsupported dictum that 'the camera never lies'.

Images are both sources (of meaning or evidence) and *resources*, in the sense that they may be deployed to convey particular impressions. The cheap portable camera means that nowadays most people include snapshots among their biographical and family archives. Such material needs to be subjected to the same careful scrutiny as publicly accessible sources, for, as Spence and others have shown in their experiments in 'photo-therapy', conventional imagery is highly selective, promoting happy moments while rendering problems invisible (Spence and Holland 1991). Photo-journalism and documentary photography, photography as art, advertising and illustration use images in different ways, each needing critical attention. Alternatively, we might also use photographs 'to answer questions the photographer did not have in mind and that are not obviously suggested by the picture . . . We can thus avoid interminable, unresolvable, and irrelevant questions about the photographer's intent' (Becker 1986: 277).

We have analysed elsewhere the stereotyping of older people through different versions of visual shorthand – cartoons, political propaganda, postcards, popular magazines (Blaikie and Macnicol 1986; Featherstone and Hepworth 1995). These studies suggest that, during the earlier twentieth century, modernity produced an enhanced awareness of stigma via the growing administrative classification of older people as a chronologically determined social group with a fixed identity; hence a gallery of figures, such as the decrepit pensioner and the benign granny. Latterly, however, the growth of consumer culture has led to the emergence of a postmodern life course accentuating a range of possible lifestyle choices. Advertising photographs both reflect and create social trends, with 'positive' ageing images increasingly to the fore. Here, however, we focus not on popular culture, but on photography as art. Two aspects are considered: first, the perceived role of images of age within the broader frame of the general photographic exhibition; second, the creative uses of photography to convey messages about ageing.

### Pictures at an exhibition

In 1994, the Barbican staged a major exhibition from the massive Hulton Deutsch Collection, entitled 'All Human Life'. Older people were not particularly predominant among the several hundred photographs on show, yet both the leaflet and the catalogue accompanying the exhibition featured them heavily. The front cover of the latter presented a close-up shot, taken in 1939, of a couple celebrating their Golden Wedding with a kiss (Bernard 1994). Meanwhile, the free leaflet portrayed 'Old Tom' Owen having his head shaved. The justification for selecting these two images – from a total of no less than 15 million in the collection – is provided in the text which introduces the catalogue: 'Amongst my own personal favourites are pictures of some of the old characters who you might still, if you are fortunate enough, stumble across every now and again . . . people like old Tom Owen, the hedge-laying specialist, loving every moment of his haircut' (Bernard 1994: 9). Here the scarcity of 'old characters', still to be 'stumbled across' on occasion, like antique stoves still in use, or classic cars, constitutes their appeal. However, the emphasis on ageing suggests a more general phenomenon.

Presenting 254 images from 27 countries, the 133rd International Exhibition of the Edinburgh Photographic Society reflected the conventional cross-section of image categories: exotic shots of faraway places, pictorial allegories with titles such as *Temptation* and *Isolation*, portraits, street and domestic scenes. Only 15 (6 per cent) of these photographs showed older people or relations between generations, yet of the 28 plates in the accompanying catalogue, five are of older people. Interestingly, another five feature children, suggesting perhaps an editorial desire to balance the two ends of the life span (Edinburgh Photographic Society 1995). Similarly, when distinguished Scots selected their seven favourite images from the National Photography Collection, older people featured in three of the chosen pictures (and 'pastness' characterizes the Victorian fisher children, and Victorian street scenes in two of the remaining four). While artist John Bellany chose an early (1844) Hill and Adamson calotype of a fishwife because 'it has the stillness and silent beauty of a Vermeer', he adds, 'Perhaps more importantly I love it because it reminds me of my Auntie Nan who used to carry the creel.' Pop musician Donnie Munro selected Iain Stewart's *Grandmother and Child*, remarking that 'It's almost like the potential of youth set against a reflective image of old age.' Finally, the Bishop of Edinburgh elected Grace Robertson's *Mother's Day Off* (1954), which depicts a young girl spying into a pub window, while in the foreground an old lady engages the attention of two middle-aged women. This picture is part of a documentary photo-essay illustrating a bus outing to Clapham Common. Bishop Holloway recollects 'grannies going down for a glass of port to the Cosy Corner'. His final comment – 'I'm sorry to give you a piece of autobiographical social history but that would be the picture I would choose' – reflects the salience of images that relate to or suggest a link with one's own past. This active biographical personalization of photographs clearly has the effect of foregrounding images of 'pastness' (rather than the present), of people (rather than buildings or landscapes) and, in particular, of people who trigger memories of childhood (National Galleries of Scotland 1994). These images also assert mortality as a central theme of photography. As Roland Barthes has observed, photographs must remind us of death since they can only ever illustrate that which has passed and gone forever. Images of old people are valuable precisely because the camera has captured them for posterity, immortalized their memory.

Such impressionistic analysis indicates an often inadvertent, but none the less socially constructed imagery of the life course. However, photography as a form of art involves processes that are more readily deconstructive than reconstructive: the diversity of identities and relations between generations is emphasized, rather than any stereotypical characteristics of ageing.

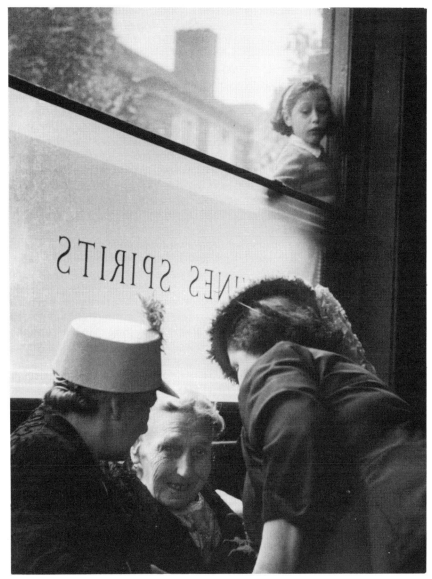

Grace Robertson, 'Mother's Day Off', 1954, Battersea. From a Picture Post photo-essay, courtesy of Zelda Cheatle Gallery, London.

## Postmodern photography: juxtaposing generations

The family is a crucial constituent in a great many photographs. Indeed, in 1994 the massively popular 'Who's Looking at the Family?' exhibition contained a number of significant works with an ageing theme (discussed in Blaikie 1995).

Each of these addressed different ways of presenting and reading interaction within and across generations by experimenting with photographic images and techniques (Williams 1994). As Pultz remarks, 'With the demise of the belief that a photograph can present a privileged window onto reality and truth, photographers have chosen instead to make pictures that admit to being artifices' (Pultz 1995: 145). While modernist documentary photographers asserted their objectivity – one that we have been at pains to undermine – artists since the 1980s have pursued their own self-conscious involvement with their subjects. The staged exploration of family relationships has been central here, and Pultz cites Sally Mann's *Sherry and Sherry's Grandmother Both at Twleve Years Old*, which poses the body of Sherry beside a cracked old photograph of her grandmother: 'Both women are represented at the age of twelve. The cultural changes in the fifty or so years that intervene between the two photographs have redefined both photography and adolescence. Unlike the dress that Sherry's grandmother wears, which is delicate and concealing, Sherry's shorts are brief, tight, and reveal[ing]' (Pultz 1995: 145).

Two recent British exhibitions similarly attempt to engage the audience in biographical exploration through juxtaposition of intergenerational images. Steven MacLaurin's installation 'They Saw My Age and Not Myself' (premiered in October 1995) encourages viewers to consider their own ageing and attitudes towards older people. On a high wall, five television screens project a series of shifting narratives, at any one moment featuring simultaneously: mother and children at the seaside in the 1940s, in bathing costumes; a sunny street scene with father and children; a wedding couple, c.1930; a young woman holding a puppy; a team photo, from schooldays. As each series gradually rotates to present further images, on the floor in front are projected five life-sized images of older women. Viewers cannot but connect the running biographies on the TV screens (like family albums) with the figures projected on the ground where they stand, but they are left to establish correspondences between one set of images and another, to imagine which snapshots 'belong' to which person's life.

Colin Gray's 'The Parents' 'is the fruit of a fifteen year project documenting the artist's own parents, reflecting upon domestic ritual, the waning of sexual desire, failing health and old age' (*Art News* September 1995). It is presented in three distinct sections. The first, Narratives, consists of theatrical tableaux of 'suburban surrealism' developed from Gray's fantasies, but staged with his parents' active collaboration and 'resonant with the new found freedom of early retirement' – for example, dressing up as Father Christmas and the Fairy Godmother in their own lounge. Such staging, according to Gray, 'arose from the need to go beyond the limits of documentary': family portraits, he feels, only serve to conceal realities behind a facade of 'acting naturally' (McArthur 1995). The second series, Close Ups, shifts abruptly to giant wall-size microscopic enlargements: 'comparisons between the worn-out carpets, furniture and utensils in the family home and the surface details of his parents' ageing bodies . . . which expose a hidden world of translucent skin, broken capillaries and liver marks' (*Art News* September 1995). The link to painting is revealed in the remarks of one of Gray's critics: 'Is this the warning of the Vanitas paintings in European art, that all life is mortal and all beauty passes?' (Beloff 1995).

Finally, in Scans, Gray uses magnetic resonance imaging, CAT scans and X-rays – all medical technologies – to illuminate the inside of his parents' bodies and their possessions. The progression in 'The Parents' then, is one from subjective interaction to objectified science, signifying the inevitability of physical betrayals and death, 'the disconcerting shift of dependence that affects each generation in time' (*Art News* September 1995). Such apparent mimicry of medical procedures implies the limitations of a socially constructed view of the ageing body – in the end biology becomes destiny.

As with McLaurin, so with Gray, 'reconsidering our own relationships must surely be a result' (Beloff 1995). Indeed, to the extent that Gray's Narratives dramatize his past memories, they may be 'allied to dream-work . . . a complex use of photography in the service of self-development' (Beloff 1995). In this important methodological respect, a focus on the family connects postmodern art with the uses of photographs in both therapy and reminiscence work (Age Exchange 1987; Spence and Holland 1991; Berman 1993).

Finally, a warning. In the creation of images of disabled people, David Hevey accuses photographic artists of 'enfreakment', a process of accentuating grotesqueness in order at once to enchant and repel the public. He cites Diane Arbus's deliberate exposition of physically and mentally disabled 'freaks' (Hevey 1992: 53–74). The offence he encounters is shared by several critics who have been upset by the absence of probity in photographing mentally retarded adults, who, by definition, were unable to give their informed consent beforehand. Arbus's late work on people in care institutions may have been designed to project 'symbolic specimens of otherness' (Lubbock 1995: 6), to 'parody our ideas about normal' by dressing up residents in Halloween masks or posing them in invented family snapshots, but the ethical transgression remains: 'Her "freaks" here do not know they are freaks and do not know there is a game going on' (Freely 1995: 16). Here art finds parallels with documentary photography, and, as Johnson and Bytheway demonstrate in this volume, such practice and critique have clear resonances when applied to the depiction of older people in institutional settings, especially those affected by mental or physical disabilities – see, for example, the photo-essay in Peter Townsend's *The Last Refuge* (1962), or the facial images of Alzheimer's sufferers depicted by Corinne Noordenbos (Williams 1994: 98–100).

Painters and photographers pose subjects according to the way they think they ought to look rather than how they are in everyday life. Regardless of whether or not we approve, both construct and reproduce ideals, be they of graceful or positive old age, happy family life, benign contentment, senility or the grotesque. They can never simply capture reality. It follows that our task must be to deconstruct their conceits, while taking care not to build our own follies.

## Acknowledgements

Andrew Blaikie wishes to acknowledge the support of the Nuffield Foundation in providing grant funding to visit and analyse photographic collections.

## References

Age Exchange (1987) *Lifetimes: a Handbook of Memories and Ideas for Use with Age Exchange Reminiscence Pictures*. London: Age Exchange.
Bartram, M. (1985) *The Pre-Raphaelite Camera: Aspects of Victorian Photography*. London: Weidenfeld and Nicolson.
Becker, H.S. (1986) Do photographs tell the truth?, in H.S. Becker (ed.) *Doing Things Together: Selected Papers*. Evanston, IL: Northwestern University Press, 273–92.
Beloff, H. (1995) Family contradictions, in C. Gray (ed.) *The Parents*. Edinburgh: Fotofeis Ltd.
Bendiner, K. (1985) *An Introduction to Victorian Painting*. New Haven, CT, and London: Yale University Press.
Berger, J. (1972) *Ways of Seeing*. Harmondsworth: BBC/Penguin.
Berman, L. (1993) *Beyond the Smile: the Therapeutic Use of the Photograph*. London: Routledge.
Bernard, B. (1994) *All Human Life: Great Photographs from the Hulton Deutsch Collection*. London: Barbican Art Gallery.
Blaikie, A. (1994) Photographic memory, ageing and the life course, *Ageing and Society*, 14(4), 479–97.
Blaikie, A. (1995) Photographic images of age and generation, *Education and Ageing*, 10(1), 5–15.
Blaikie, A. and Macnicol, J. (1986) Towards an anatomy of ageism: society, social policy and the elderly between the wars, in C. Phillipson, M. Bernard and P. Strang (eds) *Dependency and Interdependency in Old Age: Theoretical Perspectives and Policy Alternatives*. London: Croom Helm, 95–104.
Bolton, R. (1992) In the American east: Richard Avedon Incorporated, in R. Bolton (ed.) *The Contest of Meaning: Critical Histories of Photography*. London: MIT Press, 261–82.
Cowling, M. (1989) *The Artist as Anthropologist: the Representation of Type and Character in Victorian Art*. Cambridge: Cambridge University Press.
Desmond, A. and Moore, J. (1992) *Darwin*. Harmondsworth: Penguin.
Edinburgh Photographic Society (1995) *133rd International Exhibition of Photography*. Edinburgh: Edinburgh Photographic Society.
Eisenman, S.F. (1994) Introduction, in S.F. Eisenman, T. Crow, B. Lukacher, L. Nochlin and F.K. Pohl (eds) *Nineteenth Century Art: a Critical History*. London: Thames & Hudson.
Featherstone, M. and Hepworth, M. (1995) Images of positive ageing: a case study of *Retirement Choice* magazine, in M. Featherstone and A. Wernick (eds) *Images of Ageing: Cultural Representations of Later Life*. London: Routledge, 29–47.
Featherstone, M. and Hepworth, M. (1996) Images of ageing, in J. Birren *et al.* (eds) *Encyclopaedia of Gerontology, vol. 1*. San Diego: Academic Press, 743–51.
Featherstone, M. and Wernick, A. (1995) Introduction, in M. Featherstone and A. Wernick (eds) *Images of Ageing: Cultural Representations of Later Life*. London: Routledge, 1–15.
Fox, C. and Greenacre, F. (1979) *Artists of the Newlyn School 1880–1900*. Newlyn: Newlyn Orion Art Galleries.
Freely, M. (1995) At the limit of exposure, *The Guardian*, 29 September.
Hepworth, M. (1995a) Where do grannies come from?, *Generations Review*, 5(1), 2–4.
Hepworth, M. (1995b) Positive ageing: what is the message?, in R. Bunton *et al.* (eds) *The Sociology of Health Promotion: Critical Analyses of Consumption, Lifestyle and Risk*. London: Routledge, 176–90.
Hepworth, M. (1995c) Images of old age, in J. Coupland and J. Nussbaum (eds) *Handbook of Communication and Ageing Research*. New York: Erlbaum, 5–37.
Hepworth, M. (1995d) 'Wrinkles of vice and wrinkles of virtue': the moral interpretation of the ageing body, in C. Hummel *et al.* (eds) *Images of Ageing in Western Societies*. Geneva: University of Geneva Centre For Interdisciplinary Gerontology, 39–68.

Hevey, D. (1992) *The Creatures Time Forgot: Photography and Disability Imagery*. London: Routledge.

Holdsworth, S. and Crossley, J. (1992) *Innocence and Experience: Images of Children in British Art from 1660 to the Present*. Manchester: Manchester City Art Galleries.

Kay, S. and Rubin, M. (1994) Introduction, in S. Kay and M. Rubin (eds) *Framing Medieval Bodies*. Manchester and New York: Manchester University Press, 1–9.

Lister, R. (1966) *Victorian Narrative Paintings*. London: Museum Press.

Lowenthal, D. (1985) *The Past Is a Foreign Country*. Cambridge: Cambridge University Press.

Lubbock, T. (1995) More trick than treat, *The Observer Review*, 17 September.

McArthur, E. (1995) Text, in C. Gray, *The Parents*. Edinburgh: Fotofeis Ltd.

Millar, O. (1992) *The Victorian Pictures in the Collection of Her Majesty the Queen*, 2 vols: text and plates. Cambridge: Cambridge University Press.

Morrison, J. (1989) Rural nostalgia: painting in Scotland c.1860–1880. University of St Andrews, Unpublished PhD.

National Galleries of Scotland (1994) *On Photography*. Edinburgh: Education Department of the National Galleries of Scotland.

Nochlin, L. (1990) *Realism*. Harmondsworth: Penguin.

Pointon, M. (1986) *Mulready*. London: Victoria and Albert Museum.

Pointon, M. (1993) *Hanging the Head: Portraiture and Social Formation in Eighteenth Century England*. New Haven, CT, and London: Yale University Press for the Paul Mellon Centre for Studies in British Art.

Pultz, S. (1995) *Photography and the Body*. London: Weidenfeld and Nicolson.

Sillars, S. (1995) *Visualisation in Popular Fiction 1860–1960*. London: Routledge.

Spence, J. and Holland, P. (eds) (1991) *Family Snaps: the Meanings of Domestic Photography*. London: Virago.

Townsend, P. (1962) *The Last Refuge: a Survey of Residential Institutions and Homes for the Aged in England and Wales*. London: Routledge & Kegan Paul.

Treuherz, J. (1993) *Victorian Painting*. London: Thames & Hudson.

Williams, V. (1994) *Who's Looking at the Family?* London: Barbican Art Gallery.

Williams, L. (1995) 'Corporealized observers: visual pornographies and the "carnal density of vision"', in T. Petro (ed.) *Fugitive Images: from Photography to Video*. Bloomington and Indianapolis: Indiana University Press.

Zeri, F. (1990) *Behind the Image: the Art of Reading Paintings*. London: Heinemann.

# Citizenship theory and old age: from social rights to surveillance

Contemporary citizenship theory has been inextricably linked to the nature and future of welfare states since the ground breaking work of T.H. Marshall in the 1950s. The role played by the needs of older people has also been of crucial importance to this issue, given that state expenditure on this section of the population has always been considerable and seems likely to rise. This chapter looks at contemporary accounts of citizenship in the light of an ageing population and within the context of changing welfare policies. It will argue that conventional accounts of citizenship have led the structural dependency school of social gerontologists to argue that older people have had full citizenship rights denied to them. This in turn dominates the analysis and proposed solutions offered by the approach. The growing importance of consumption and lifestyle in modern social life undermines many of the assumptions central to citizenship theory and practice and necessitates a revision of the usefulness of the concept. The chapter will therefore also look at how more contemporary accounts of citizenship, advanced in particular by Bryan Turner and Anthony Giddens, have tried to incorporate these developments, and how increasingly they come to focus on the issue of the state's relation to old age. Taking a different approach, I will suggest that citizenship should be viewed in terms of the surveillance of older people rather than an articulation of their rights.[1]

## Citizenship and the welfare state

T.H. Marshall's model of citizenship (Marshall 1992) is widely known and is seen as providing a basis for integrating individuals and classes with the wider community. Written in 1950, it was an optimistic formulation based on the idea that in Britain there had been a historical progression of freedom, moving from civil to social rights between the eighteenth and twentieth centuries. That post-war Britain represented the triumph of social development was taken as read (Titmuss 1974). The inequalities created through the industrial revolution and the market were to be contained by the state in order to establish social harmony. Citizens were to have a stake in society; one which removed the desire to change radically the institutional order or challenge the centrality of the market. It is important to note that Marshall's account of citizenship was not just a theory, but rather was a justification of the strategy pursued by post-war governments, who were to pursue policies dedicated to egalitarian collectivist ends.

The full title of Marshall's *Citizenship and Social Class* is significant, because it highlights his view that the development of capitalist society creates profound class inequality. This in turn provides opportunities for political radicalism to undermine social stability. To ensure that social inequality was reduced, Marshall pointed to a secondary system of industrial citizenship created by the trade unions, which through collective bargaining could act as an instrument for raising workers' social and economic status and thus promote social unity. In this way, civil rights which were individualistic could turn into collective social rights. Added to this was the impact of welfare policies and progressive taxation, which modified the whole pattern of social inequality and subordinated market relations to social justice.

A range of theoretical criticisms have been directed at Marshall's account of citizenship, centring on issues such as its historical accuracy (Rees 1996), its Anglo-centrism (Mann 1987) and its failure to acknowledge the importance of conflict (Giddens 1982). Of probably more importance is the failure to see the gendering of citizenship that was implicit in the original design (Pedersen 1993) so that women fail to have their social needs established as rights. The conflation of nationality with citizenship is another aspect of Marshall's account that was seemingly unproblematic at the time but which has become of central concern to politics since the 1960s (Rees 1996).

At a more pragmatic level, the strategy of citizenship has been remarkably unsuccessful in achieving its ends, in that it led to neither class abatement nor social justice. The heyday of citizenship theory and practice occurred at a time when the majority of the population was clearly stratified into the defined occupational groups of a mass society (Cronin 1984) where class interests could be identified and appealed to. Marshall's idea of social equality responded to such a world by offering mass benefits and mass entitlements. The vision was successful but the reality not always so. As with nationalization, the social effectiveness of the Keynesian welfare state did not always live up to its potential. Class inequalities remained and often widened. On top of this, those who received maximum benefit from the new structures were often middle class, both through employment and through increased opportunity (Le Grand 1982).

More significantly, at the point during the 1970s when economic recession made the claims of citizenship practical, what was on offer was dramatically reduced. Instead of offering a safety net against the degrading effects of market instability, the welfare state was used as a structure of labour discipline (Gough 1979). The benefits in kind that made up the social wage were also reduced and, indeed, blamed for the poor state the economy was in in the first place (Taylor-Gooby 1991).

These new circumstances made belief in what had always been a contradictory ideal of citizenship difficult (Higgs 1993), particularly as they were accompanied by successive incomes policies which cut deeply into the living standards of the then still relatively cohesive organized working class (Kavanagh 1990). In part, this state of affairs could be attributed to some of the instabilities that existed within Marshall's account of the relationship between capitalism and social class (Hindess 1993). The compromise (or stand-off) could not last indefinitely, and Hindess points to the use of the term hyphenated society to describe a 'democratic-welfare-capitalism' in Marshall's later work.

## The decline of citizenship

A more fundamental undermining of both the theory and practice of citizenship emerged with the resurgence of economic neo-liberalism in the 1970s and 1980s. To the 'new right' the social rights embodied in citizenship were seen as anathema. The rights of citizenship led to bureaucracy, inefficiency and the power of the state over all individuals. Furthermore, it led to economic stagnation and decline as the leviathan of the expanding public purse crushed all initiative through taxation and regulation (Kymlicka and Norman 1994). The policies followed by the Thatcher government in the UK and the Reagan administration in the USA can be seen as deliberate attempts to limit social citizenship; however, some commentators have argued that the changes represent appropriate responses to the changing nature of society.

Peter Saunders (1993) argues that such moves do not undermine citizenship but instead promote it. It is no longer true that a considerable proportion of the working population does not receive enough wages to cover its own reproduction. Consequently the need for the 'socialized consumption' of state welfare has declined as real incomes have risen. This affluence as well as the increased cost of welfare has resulted in a shift to 'privatized consumption', where being a purchaser of services is as important as questions of quality and choice. As an example of this shift, he points to the popularity of the sale of council houses by the Conservative government during the 1980s. This differentiation also has its effects on those left behind, who are likely to become dissatisfied as they compare their relative fate with those able to privatize their consumption.

Zygmunt Bauman (1988), from a different political position, makes the same point about being a recipient of state welfare. In an era characterized by consumption and choice, people use commodities to establish their self-identities. Those who do not have the resources to participate in the market become 'repressed' welfare clients subject to the controlling disciplinary mechanisms of the state. While not everyone would accord with this view of the 'sovereign consumer' (Warde 1994), what does seem to be true is the general acceptance of the inferiority of state welfare: so much so that supporters of the Marshallian idea of citizenship have accepted that there was much wrong with the welfare state, especially in its lack of respect for individuals and its concentration on 'statist' solutions or in its reliance on corporatism (Ferris 1985; Plant 1988). Consequently, at both a theoretical and a practical level there has been an abandonment of the conventional idea of citizenship.

## Structured dependency theory and citizenship

Structured dependency theory has been the dominant trend in British social gerontology since the 1980s, and has implicitly adopted a citizenship strategy for older people. The approach argues that the dependent social position of older people is a direct effect of social policy (Townsend 1981). Attention is directed to pension arrangements, employment practices and discriminatory health policies. These in turn create environments where older people are excluded, marginalized or infantilized. As a consequence, it is ageism not biology that dominates the lives of most older people. The problems that older people face in Britain are consequently ones that can be overcome by determined policy and through realizing the full possibilities of citizenship.

Social gerontologists have made strenuous efforts to separate the idea of old age from the processes of ill-health and physical frailty because this allows social gerontology to stress the similarities that exist across the generations and challenge the cultural assumptions of generational discontinuity (Arber and Evandrou 1993). In claiming that older people are not a homogeneous group linked together by a common physical frailty and that retired people are as diverse as the rest of the population, scope has been provided for the idea of an active old age. However, a major limiting factor is the low level of the state retirement pension, which provides pensioners with only a small proportion of the average wage (Townsend 1981; Townsend and Walker 1995), and it is a proportion that is likely to decrease further (Evandrou and Falkingham 1993). In identifying this issue, an explicit political strategy of advocating full citizenship rights for older people emerges.

Phillipson (1982) has argued that these rights need to be organized, so that exclusion from the wage economy does not itself lead older people into an inferior social category. Other rights can vary in scope from anti-age discriminatory legislation to the creation of representative political structures. Generally, however, they prioritize the need for a radical reworking of pensions policy if greater equality is to be created. In a *Manifesto for Old Age*, Bornat *et al.* (1985) propose that the 'retirement pension needs to be greatly increased, to a level which provides a "participation standard" of living for all pensioners. This would probably be higher than the pensioner movement's current goal of one-third the average wage for a single person' (Bornat *et al.* 1985: 78–9). In this way, one of the fundamental social rights of citizenship would be established. Laczko and Phillipson (1991) also point to the importance of reworking pensions policy by abandoning the traditional work/retirement dichotomy through the introduction of a 'decade of retirement', with much greater flexibility for workers wanting to leave employment gradually but without negative financial effects in the shape of lower pensions. More recently, Townsend and Walker (1995) have made an explicit appeal for both a return to a universalist pensions policy and an uprating of benefit rates.

Creating the basis for an active participation in society through financial means also provides the basis for a reordering of the relationship between older people and health. The stereotyping of old age as infirmity would be challenged as active older people become visible in society. Where physical infirmity or chronic illness did arise, older people would be able to utilize their position within the community to make decisions about what older people themselves wanted. All in all, what many different writers are describing is the full integration of older people into society rather than an acceptance of their disengagement or separateness; a position adopted by an earlier (American) tradition (Cummings and Henry 1964). Integrating old age into a concept of a life course shared by all humans benefits not only older people but also those of different generations. As Arber and Ginn (1991) have argued, much feminist research has concentrated on the gendered nature of informal care of older people. On occasion this focus has seemingly produced a division of interest between younger women carers and the older people being cared for. One strand of the manifesto advocated by Bornat *et al.* attempts to minimize these conflicts through the creation and funding of formalized caring options and support.

A major difficulty with the citizenship approach is that in trying to overcome structured dependency, many of the proposals end up homogenizing all older people into an undifferentiated group who need to be made equal. This is not surprising given that the idea of citizenship being used is one that still works from the assumption of mass benefits. As a result, the recognition that structural inequalities in old age are often the effects of earlier social differences leads *A Manifesto for Old Age* to advocate the limiting of certain privileges associated with occupational pensions. A similar effect is produced by many of the studies examining income differences in old age. The poverty of large proportions of older people is identified, while effectively erasing the existence of more affluent sections of the older population. Even when it is acknowledged that this group exists and is likely to increase in the future, the full implications are not considered (Wilson 1993). Pointing out the relative affluence of many older people does not mean that poverty is not important among large numbers of older people; rather, it establishes the point that approaches based on structured dependency theory are almost obliged to adopt a welfarist approach to old age. That there are limitations to this view can be gleaned from the fact that government social policy seems not to be interested in overcoming structured dependency and that older people themselves don't seem to be motivated by the issue (Ginn 1994). Another significant problem is that the approach has difficulties dealing with the realities of older people who see old age from the perspective of lifestyle. These 'third agers' seem to give the lie to many of the tenets of structured dependency by constructing old age as a process of leisure (Featherstone and Hepworth 1986, 1991; Laslett 1989). Though possibly limited in numbers, it is likely that succeeding generations of older people are more likely to see themselves from this perspective – rather than as old age trade unionists. It is interesting to note that Laczko and Phillipson (1991) are aware of these developments but feel constrained to look to policy and debate to 'develop the vision of what life in retirement could be about' (Laczko and Phillipson 1991: 129) rather than accept that it is already happening. The limitations of structured dependency theory are therefore twofold: it adopts a stance which sees the position of older people as ultimately homogeneous and powerless; and it assumes that it is only through mass social benefits that any improvement can occur. Both of these positions are erroneous and inhibit the objectives of social gerontology. Not only has the conventional view of citizenship been seen to fail in practice, it is also theoretically flawed.

## The state, status and citizenship

An alternative to the social democratic view of citizenship and old age has been developed by Bryan Turner (1988, 1989, 1990, 1993). Acknowledging that Marshall's approach was culturally bound to the shores of Britain and that it was unproblematically teleological, Turner counters that citizenship is intrinsically bound up in the nature of modern society. As the highly stratified social structures of Western industrialized capitalism give way to the more fragmented forms of consumer society, so the importance of status increases (Turner 1988: 43–78). Status has the power to include or exclude individuals from a community or society. So has citizenship. In this way citizenship is a form of status which is based upon being a full member of a modern nation state. At its most conventional, Turner is adopting Parsons's ideas regarding the civil rights struggles in America. For black people in the USA, their exclusion from the 'public sphere' indicated, if not created, a lack of status and therefore of power. To be a citizen and to be accepted as one is therefore extremely important in the social construction of groups.

Turner goes further, and argues that as traditional occupational structures play less and less of a role in most people's day-to-day activities, a multitude of lifestyle choices come to replace them. Status politics based around group identities become crucial as the practicalities of policy formation and implementation in the public sphere. Unlike in the work of Max Weber, the politics of Turner's status groups are played out in the realm of the welfare state or in the grey area of the state-assisted voluntary organization. To extend Turner's argument, it would seem that the collapse of the salience of class in society is reflected in the rejection of mass provision of welfare. This does not diminish the idea of citizenship, because status groups primarily want their particular needs met and may be unconcerned as to the form in which they are. It could be further argued that a more flexible welfare environment would be more responsive to them than powerful welfare bureaucracies. Special interests perspectives and budgetary control over resources might go a long way in weakening the hold of a universalistic, public sector dominated, mass welfare system.

Older people are, according to Turner, in competition with other social groups because the negative experience of ageing results in them being denied their universalistic rights of citizenship. This leads Turner to describe them as a 'state administered status group', because they become the clients of the state in order to enforce their social entitlements (Turner 1989: 592). Turner clearly sees the possibility of the development of a politics of old age in the mould of the US 'Gray Panthers', because, he argues, 'competitive struggle between social groups over resources [is] the essential feature of a sociology of status' (Turner 1989: 593). Such competition has the effect of creating social solidarity and identity within the group. The consequence of this, according to Turner, is not a threat to social cohesion but rather an extension of social membership, as conflict provides a way in which enhanced social mobility will be possible, at least in principle. He writes:

> My view of status conflicts is in this limited sense 'positive', since I treat this competitive struggle as a process which brings about various forms of social solidarity and group membership. Social welfare rights as a consequence of political struggle are also mechanisms for the integration of oppositional and marginal groups within the political community. Inflationary wage spirals may be unintentionally a safety valve against more violent forms of political protest.
>
> (Turner 1989: 593)

Running through Turner's argument is the notion of active citizenship, which can only take shape in relation to the nature of the state. Marshall's argument is criticized for not having a clear theory of the state. This is important because, following Mann (1987), the policies adopted by a state dictate the form citizenship will take. Mann outlines five differing ruling class strategies. All of them involve deliberate attempts to deal with modernity and industrialization, and most significantly the political threat represented by the working class. A consequence of this is whether or not citizens are active or passive and whether the individual's concerns are strictly private or whether they can be addressed in the public realm. Certain formations allow for the development of an active citizenry, such as revolutionary French tradition, and some do not, such as the German experience of fascism. The public sphere is either open as in Britain or closed as in the USA.

Taking this extension of Turner's argument, it would seem that if the concept of citizenship and old age is to mean anything it has to be based on both a notion of public activism and a public sphere in which to act. These two conditions seem to be questionable, at least in current circumstances. A further problem is the fact that older citizens, active or not, are presented as one of the causes of social crisis through their disproportionate demands for welfare resources (Thomson 1989). Such inter-generational conflicts lead, at least in principle, to more than just interest group competition.

Turner's (1993) more recent work provides further examples of this difficulty, in that it relies on an acceptance of social rights in the public arena. Stemming from Turner's interest in postmodernism, he has moved his analysis on to look at what happens in the more culturally fragmented environment of globalization, where the nation state has lost a considerable amount of its power. Relating to the growth of such bodies as the European Union, he argues that the repository of social rights has to move to pan-national entities such as this if they are to have any meaning. Such post-national citizenship will have to be based increasingly on ideas of European identity, in which no specific culture can be articulated. Instead, Turner sees the multiplicity of cultural identities all receiving their legitimacy from their respect for one another, and all enshrined in human rights. What Turner posits as 'cultural citizenship' is based on what he calls the democratization of culture which a fragmentary postmodern culture has now made possible. Returning to a theme of Marshall's – that an active citizen must be capable of sharing in a common culture in order fully to participate in society – Turner argues that the collapse of the distinction between high and low culture allows all citizens to do precisely that. No particular set of ideas can dominate and difference must be accepted. As Roche (1995) has pointed out, there is a deep acknowledged ambivalence in Turner's work about how the nation state based concept of citizenship meshes with postmodern cultural fragmentation, and whether the latter will make the former redundant. Roche himself feels that such transnational citizenship is unlikely to be achieved, partly because such bodies as the EU do not have the capacity to grant citizenship themselves but must establish it through one of the member states first, and are therefore subordinate to them. The strategy of gaining Euro-rights for older people is thus also limited in its effectiveness. Mobilizing strategies such as the 'European Year of Older People and Solidarity between the Generations' might act as a focus for awareness, but are ultimately constrained by the Europe-wide concern about an ageing society.

At this juncture, it is interesting to note the comments made in the recent work of Anthony Giddens (1994) regarding old age and what he terms 'positive welfare'. He starts by reaffirming many of the points already outlined in this chapter about the failure of the welfare state and the individualism of modern social life. Linking these concerns with Ulrich Beck's (1992) concept of 'risk society', he argues that whereas for the purposes of the welfare state the risk that individuals were subjected to could be calculated and provision made for, under the new circumstances of reflexive modernization all of us are exposed to 'manufactured risk', which cannot. This new reality is a product of both the tremendous unintended consequences of industrialization and the growing incapacity of knowledge to anticipate or adequately explain them. The ageing of the population, argues Giddens, must be seen from this perspective. Making many of the points familiar to social gerontologists, he points out the negative social impact of being a pensioner, but crucially argues: 'Ageing is treated as "external", as something that happens to one, not as a phenomenon actively constructed and negotiated' (Giddens 1994: 170). Giddens sees the future of old age as being to remove this external label and make older persons more constitutive of themselves. In practice, this means taking more responsibility for individual health as well as removing the state pension as an unnecessary form of 'precautionary aftercare', with the intention of creating the 'autotelic self' who not only has self-respect and ontological security but also challenges risk as a way of achieving self-actualization. Obviously this is challenging stuff as far as contemporary politics is concerned, but it is flawed by the collapsing of structure into agency, which is a criticism made of structuration theory (Callinicos 1985). Either way, the concept of citizenship disappears into the autotelic self.

The work of Turner and Giddens suggests that holding on to a notion of old age and citizenship while discarding its universalist collectivist underpinnings dislocates the usefulness of the term as far as social gerontology is concerned.

## Citizenship as surveillance

Given the dilemmas about the viability of the idea of citizenship outlined above, it may be more useful to confine the concept to the issue of procedural rights for individuals and drop the foundation of collective or mass substantive rights. Present social policy in Britain seems to be going in this direction. The Citizen's Charter is an ideal, building on various specific charters in health, railways and government. Citizenship in this form is a relationship between the state and the individual. The citizen can expect to be treated in certain ways and can reasonably expect specified levels of service. Treatment that does not meet these standards can be complained about and compensation secured. This provides the basis of a model which may be more realistic as well as more theoretically fruitful.

Implicit in this model is the idea of contract. This cornerstone of civil law is applied not only positively to members of the public dealing with large public and private sector organizations but also negatively to those receiving welfare benefits. For example, unemployed people seeking the 'jobseeker's allowance' now make a formal contract to undertake certain job-seeking activities, such as regularly going to a job centre or applying for a specified number of jobs every week. The idea of entitlement as conceived by Marshall has been replaced by a 'bourgeois' concept of contract. The use of the Social Fund exemplifies this approach, where ability to pay back a 'loan' is an equal criterion for entitlement with need.

Contracts are also expected to dominate at an institutional level. Health authorities are expected to purchase an appropriate range of health services on behalf of individuals in their local populations; that is, if fundholding general practices are not already doing so. Likewise, social services departments are expected to set contracts for individually tailored packages of community care. In both of these cases, individuals have their needs assessed and met by organizations acting on their behalf. Rights and obligations are also invested by individuals in these organizations, against whom complaints can be taken out and expectations made.

As can be seen, individuation is the starting point of this new reworking of the idea of citizenship. As such, it reflects aspects that have always been present in civil society: the importance of contract, equality of treatment, freedom of choice etc. (Green 1993). It would be a mistake, however, to view these changes as simply the return to the *laissez-faire* social policies of the Victorian era. Rather than being a retreat from the welfare state, it represents a change in the organizing principle of state welfare.

At the centre of this change is the notion of the abstract individual that exists in civil society and which modern social policy is increasingly moving towards. However, this is more than just the 'docile body' subject to disciplinary power that Foucault (1979) was writing about. The model citizen is a composite of norms, values and statistics against which real ones are measured and assessed. Deviations from this frame of reference are then the appropriate subject of social policy, which is fundamentally concerned with how to get individuals back to conforming to this model or, if this fails, or is impossible, with how to exclude and control the particular deviant individual or group. Armstrong (1995) has talked of the emergence of what he terms 'surveillance medicine', where the whole of the individual's life is subject to scrutiny for risky behaviours that might give rise to future health problems. This process does not just exist at a medical level or indeed just for adults, it also relates to education, social services and disability (Hewitt 1992). Children are now routinely monitored through national testing, through the health services and through the welfare services. In each of these areas, expert derived concepts of normality or appropriateness are utilized and those individuals causing concern by not meeting them are given special attention. This is not to argue that what is noted has no value or is done with sinister intentions, but rather that it sees the individual as a version of the normal, however that is defined.

According to Giddens (1985), surveillance of the population is central to the activities of the modern nation state, given that with larger populations direct repressive power is more and more difficult to organize. Giddens's development of the work of Michel Foucault is acknowledged. Even more relevant is Foucault's idea of 'governmentality' (Foucault 1991), which can be extended to inform the current debates about citizenship and older people. This concept refers to the ordering of populations around particular ideas or discourses, with the object of administering them. Again, the process concentrates on abstract factors and not concrete individuals. Castel (1991) argues that populations are monitored in terms of risk: 'A risk does not arise from the presence of a particular precise danger embodied in a concrete individual or group. It is the effect of a combination of abstract "factors" which render more or less probable the occurrence of undesirable modes of behaviour' (Castel 1991: 287). The current interest in health promotion and AIDS surveillance can be seen as examples of this.

The implications of governmentality for the state are immense. If the organization of welfare can be understood as a technical problem of risk avoidance, then the nature of state welfare can be radically rearranged. Assessment and administration become the main if not the only functions of the welfare state. As Castel points out, in an era of state welfare contraction 'the interventionist technologies which make it possible to "guide" and "assign" individuals without having to assume their custody could well prove to be a decisive resource' (Castel 1991: 295).

Following this line of argument, it could be argued that old age is being treated in this technical fashion. As mentioned above, the state pension is extremely important for many older people in the UK, but whether this is likely to remain so is debatable. In Britain, pensions policy is focused around the growing numbers with occupational or private pensions, leaving the state pension as a concern only of a minority. Increasingly, the idea that universal pensions 'waste' money on those who don't need it allows a more differentiated idea of welfare to emerge. Targeting those who are in greatest need is therefore a technical solution which promotes individuality and, arguably, provides better resources for those in need. This does not mean that resources are not being allocated to older people; they are, but not as part of a universalist welfare programme. Older people benefit in different ways depending on their status and their resources. A further advantage of such a policy is the separating out of a group of older people as primarily welfare benefit recipients among a population of self-supporting, self-reliant older people. In this way, the ideal of the citizen as consumer relates to both the discourse of modern life and individual reality. What is more, according to Hewitt (1996), if self-reliance was compulsory such a course of action could also help the economy through investment. As a model she has in mind the way the Singapore government utilizes its central provident fund to make individual citizens responsible for their own welfare and to invest in the economy.

The relevance of governmentality to health care and citizenship is also apparent. In health care older people are presented with two images; one is physically frail and dependent while the other is active and healthy, a third ager. Ironically, the new rights of citizenship provided by the reforms to health and social services relate to the first, while only being meaningful to the second. The ability to exercise choice depends on there being an active consumer who is able to make informed and real decisions. Frailty and dependency are not ideal circumstances from which to exercise consumer sovereignty. Power imbalances and real physical limitations are just two impediments.

This conundrum illustrates the contradictory nature of this new mode of citizenship. Citizens, through 'technologies of the self' (Foucault 1988), are encouraged to take greater personal responsibility for their health and for extending the period of their third age; however, as those who move into a fourth age of needing health and welfare services discover, at this point they are transformed from consumers into objects of consumption. The 'medical gaze' which becomes almost statutory at the age of 75 observes, investigates and regulates older people. The surveying state is at its height. Commitments to individuality made in the Patient's Charter are unlikely to overcome the fact that on an acute medical or surgical ward the old person's body is little more than an object of health care discourse:

> Old people are hurried in and out, their physical and social status assessed and their frailties noted and attended to as efficiently as possible within the law: or they lie, waiting to be claimed by some citizen consumer, a.k.a. carer, where the health service can discharge its responsibilities . . . And yet, ironically at the point when the body becomes the defining element in a person's life, the health care professionals reorientate themselves. They construct disembodied packages of care in which the fourth ager becomes a series of categories of response; a new cultural text of met and unmet need.
>
> (Gilleard and Higgs 1996: 19)

Consumer citizenship for older people depends to a great extent on their resources and health. They are continually being surveyed, but the risks have not yet mounted up to demand intervention. The rolling back of the monolithic and bureaucratic welfare state is not primarily about offering choice and freedom from the 'nanny state'. Rather, it is about acknowledging that the state doesn't have to get involved in providing responses to risk – it only needs to identify them.

Hence there is the creation of a targeted or eligible group of older people who have been designated as at risk. These form a sub-class of consumers unable to exercise choice, even though they are the only ones eligible to receive services paid for or organized by the state. This provides the modern meaning of citizenship, because the only way, it seems, to appreciate fully the fruits of citizenship is to move into the fourth age. This being the case, it is not accidental that active seniors have purposefully to separate themselves from, but live in fear of, the fourth age. Their role as citizens is comfortable so long as it is confined to their procedural rights – the substantive rights of social citizenship, on the other hand, are something to be apprehensive about. This may be why acute health care is very much a political issue in the UK and long-term institutional and community care is not.

## Conclusion

The circumstances of consumer citizenship make the likelihood of a politics of old age unlikely. The idea that older people will be able to utilize their position as consumers is as naive here as it has always been. The modern citizen is there to be monitored for 'risk', not to be active. Denial of old age by older people themselves is already more advanced as a strategy and will continue to be so. Participation in the culture of the third age is an inevitable part of the social world today, whether older people want it or not. How that culture is negotiated is the problem for all older people. In the future, the role of citizenship in this process may be limited if not redundant. Those approaching retirement as well as those experiencing it will be fully aware that its value has steadily been diminishing and any successful old age is fully their responsibility.

## Note

1  This chapter reworks some of the ideas contained in an earlier article in *Ageing and Society* (Higgs 1995).

## References

Arber, S. and Evandrou, M. (1993) Mapping the territory, in S. Arber and M. Evandrou (eds) *Ageing, Independence and the Lifecourse*. London: Jessica Kingsley.
Arber, S. and Ginn, J. (1991) The invisibility of age: gender and class in later life, *Sociological Review*, 36(1), 33–47.
Armstrong, D. (1995) The rise of surveillance medicine, *Sociology of Health and Illness*, 17(3), 393–404.
Bauman, Z. (1988) *Freedom*. Milton Keynes: Open University Press.

Beck, U. (1992) *Risk Society: towards a New Modernity*. London: Sage.

Bornat, J., Phillipson, P. and Ward, S. (1985) *A Manifesto for Old Age*. London: Pluto.

Callinicos, A. (1985) Anthony Giddens – a contemporary critique, *Theory and Society*, 14, 133–66.

Castel, R. (1991) From dangerousness to risk, in R. Burchell (ed.) *The Foucault Effect*. Hemel Hempstead: Harvester Wheatsheaf.

Cronin, J. (1984) *Labour and Society in Britain 1918–1979*. London: Batsford.

Cummings, E. and Henry, W. (1961) *Growing Old*. New York: Basic Books.

Evandrou, M. and Falkingham, J. (1993) Social security and the life course: developing sensitive policy alternatives, in S. Arber and M. Evandrou (eds) *Ageing, Independence and the Lifecourse*. London: Jessica Kingsley.

Featherstone, M. and Hepworth, M. (1986) New lifestyles in old age?, in C. Phillipson *et al.* (eds) *Dependency and Interdependency in Old Age: Theoretical Perspectives and Policy Alternatives*. Beckenham: Croom Helm.

Featherstone, M. and Hepworth, M. (1991) The mask of ageing and the postmodern life course, in M. Featherstone, M. Hepworth and B. Turner (eds) *The Body: Social Processes and Cultural Theory*. London: Sage.

Ferris, J. (1985) Citizenship and the crisis of the welfare state, in P. Bean *et al.* (eds) *In Defence of Welfare*. London: Tavistock.

Foucault, M. (1979) *The History of Sexuality, Vol. 1*. Harmondsworth: Penguin.

Foucault, M. (1988) Technologies of the self, in L. Martin, H. Gutman and P. Hutton (eds) *Technologies of the Self: a Seminar with Michel Foucault*. London: Tavistock.

Foucault, M. (1991) Governmentality, in R. Burchell (ed.) *The Foucault Effect*. Hemel Hempstead: Harvester Wheatsheaf.

Giddens, A. (1982) *Profiles and Critiques in Social Theory*. London: Macmillan.

Giddens, A. (1985) *The Nation-state and Violence*. Cambridge: Polity.

Giddens, A. (1994) *Beyond Left and Right*. Cambridge: Polity.

Gilleard, C. and Higgs, P. (1996) Cultures of ageing: self, citizen and the body, in V. Minichiello *et al.* (eds) *Sociology of Aging*. Melbourne: International Sociological Association.

Ginn, J. (1994) Grey power: age-based organisations' response to structured inequalities, *Critical Social Policy*, 28, 23–47.

Gough, I. (1979) *The Political Economy of the Welfare State*. London: Macmillan.

Green, D. (1993) *Reinventing Civil Society*. London: IEA Health and Welfare Unit.

Hewitt, B. (1992) *Welfare, Needs and Ideology*. Hemel Hempstead: Harvester Wheatsheaf.

Hewitt, P. (1996) Social justice in a global economy, in M. Bulmer and A. Rees (eds) *Citizenship Today: the Contemporary Relevance of T.H. Marshall*. London: UCL Press.

Higgs, P. (1993) *The NHS and Ideological Conflict*. Aldershot: Avebury.

Higgs, P. (1995) Citizenship and old age: the end of the road?, *Ageing and Society*, 15, 535–50.

Hindess, B. (1993) Citizenship in the modern West, in B. Turner (ed.) *Citizenship and Social Theory*. London: Sage.

Kavanagh, D. (1990) *Thatcherism and British Politics*. Oxford: Oxford University Press.

Kymlicka, W. and Norman, W. (1994) Return of the citizen: a survey of recent work on citizenship theory, *Ethics*, 104, 352–81.

Laczko, F. and Phillipson, C. (1991) *Changing Work and Retirement*. Buckingham: Open University Press.

Laslett, P. (1989) *A Fresh Map of Life: the Emergence of the Third Age*. London: Weidenfeld and Nicolson.

Le Grand, J. (1982) *The Strategy of Equality*. London: Allen and Unwin.

Leonard, P. (1982) Introduction, in P. Phillipson, *Capitalism and the Construction of Old Age*. London: Macmillan.

Mann, M. (1987) Ruling class strategies and citizenship, *Sociology*, 21, 339–54.

Marshall, T.H. (1992) *Citizenship and Social Class*. London: Pluto.

Midwinter, E. (1992) Citizenship: from ageism to participation, The Carnegie Inquiry into the Third Age, Research Paper No. 8, Dunfermline.

Pedersen, S. (1993) *Family, Dependence and the Origins of the Welfare State 1914–1945*. Cambridge: Cambridge University Press.

Phillipson, C. (1982) *Capitalism and the Construction of Old Age*. London: Macmillan.

Plant, R. (1988) *Citizenship, Rights and Socialism*. London: Fabian Society, Pamphlet No. 531.

Rees, A. (1996) T.H. Marshall and the progress of citizenship, in M. Bulmer and A. Rees (eds) *Citizenship Today: the Contemporary Relevance of T.H. Marshall*. London: UCL Press.

Roche, M. (1995) Citizenship and modernity, *British Journal of Sociology*, 46, 715–33.

Saunders, P. (1993) Citizenship in a liberal society, in B. Turner (ed.) *Citizenship and Social Theory*. London: Sage.

Taylor-Gooby, P. (1991) *Social Change, Social Welfare and Social Science*. Hemel Hempstead: Harvester Wheatsheaf.

Thomson, D. (1989) The welfare state and generation conflict, in P. Johnson *et al.* (eds) *Workers versus Pensioners*. Manchester: Manchester University Press.

Titmuss, R. (1974) *Commitment to Welfare*. London: George Allen and Unwin.

Townsend, P. (1981) The structured dependency of the elderly: a creation of social policy in the 20th century, *Ageing and Society*, 1, 5–28.

Townsend, P. and Walker, A. (1995) *The Future of Pensions: Revitalising National Insurance*. Nottingham: European Labour Forum.

Turner, B. (1988) *Status*. Buckingham: Open University Press.

Turner, B. (1989) Ageing, status politics and social theory, *British Journal of Sociology*, 40, 588–606.

Turner, B. (1990) Outline of a theory of citizenship, *Sociology*, 24, 189–217.

Turner, B. (1993) Postmodern culture/modern citizens, in B. van Steenbergen (ed.) *The Condition of Citizenship*. London: Sage.

Warde, A. (1994) Consumers, consumption and post-Fordism, in R. Burrows and B. Loader (eds) *Towards a Post-Fordist Welfare State?* London: Routledge.

Wilson, G. (1993) Money and independence in old age, in S. Arber and M. Evandrou (eds) *Ageing, Independence and the Lifecourse*. London: Jessica Kingsley.

JULIA JOHNSON AND BILL BYTHEWAY

# Illustrating care: images of care relationships with older people

## Introduction

Public images are images that are in public circulation rather than in private minds. As Featherstone and Hepworth (1993) point out, in studying cultural aspects of later life we should be interested in a 'wide array of public images which include paintings, drawings, sculptures, photographs, advertisements, films, television productions, novels and plays' (p. 304). Our focus here is on publicly available illustrations of care relationships with older people. When these are photographs, as Featherstone and Hepworth (1993: 306) argue, they have an 'immediacy and facticity which makes us think they are real and self-evident.' Hence illustrations, and in particular photographs, have a potentially powerful role to play in the cultural construction of later life and in the development of practice in care-giving.

Fifteen years ago The Open University course, 'An Ageing Population', drew attention to images of later life: the way in which a *Help the Aged* poster, for example, portrayed later life as a time of loneliness and misery and older people as being in need of pity and charity (Gearing and Slater 1979: 61). With the notable exception of Blaikie (1994), the role of photographic images in the construction of later life in the UK remains relatively unexplored. In this chapter we analyse and discuss public representations of care relationships with older people.

Our interest started with two very similar photographs, which appeared in consecutive editions of a news bulletin published by Counsel and Care, a charitable organization that provides advice and help for older people (Counsel and Care 1993, 1994) – particularly in relation to residential care. The first, by Sam Tanner, was the winning entry of a photographic competition held during the 1993 European Community 'Year of Older People and Solidarity between the Generations'. A total of 1,500 entries were submitted from across Europe. The photojournalist Grace Robertson was one of the judges. In commenting on these entries, she said, 'These are photographs that collectively reflect . . . a life enhancing concern for how we see one another' (Counsel and Care 1993). In other words, they project a specific and laudable image of the inter-generational caring relationship.

The second photograph is similarly composed, in representing an idealized image of the same caring relationship. We noted a number of features that these two photographs have in common. First, they are of women. Second, it is the older woman who is talking – both demonstratively and demonstrably as indicated by raised hands. In Evers's (1983) terms, she is portrayed as an 'active initiator' rather than a 'passive responder'. Third, the younger person is the listener, whose attentiveness and engagement is conveyed through her leaning forward and maintaining direct eye contact – in the first the younger person is holding the hand of the speaker. This presents a positive image of care and concern. The postures and expressions convey a sense of sharing and affirmation. Fourth, a sense of symmetry and equality is created through the younger person sitting at the same level and as directly opposite the older person as possible. Finally, there are smiles – a sense of happiness and fulfilment rather than pain or sadness pervades.

It is interesting that in both photographs the older people are sitting with their chairs against a wall alongside other older people. This image of the lounge in a residential care home has a long tradition, dating back to pictures

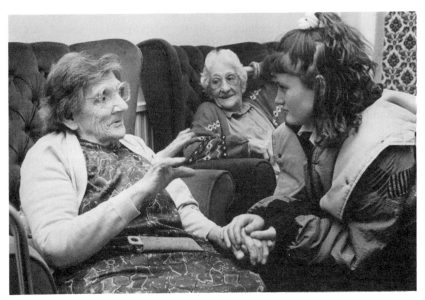

*The competition-winning entry*
Photograph: Sam Tanner

of the workhouse. It was clearly conveyed in photographs included in *The Last Refuge*, Townsend's devastating critique of residential care published in 1962, and has continued to be a familiar image of residential care, one that is commonly seen to be undesirable. This negative aspect, however, has been counteracted in the two photographs selected by Counsel and Care by the animation which generates a positive image – despite the seating arrangements. Even the occupants of the adjacent chairs are shown in a positive light: one listening to the exchange equally attentively and the other, it would seem, reading a book or newspaper. Featherstone and Hepworth (1993: 306) suggest that 'images function to invoke a particular meaning in relation to the context in which they are used, they are also symbolically charged to give expression to appropriate emotions and feeling tones.' In the context of the Counsel and Care news bulletin, the meanings that these photographs appear to invoke are: (a) that older people, including those living in residential care homes, are active and engaging people; (b) that these homes are largely occupied by older women; (c) that care is a gendered activity; and (d) that living and working in a residential care home for older people is a rewarding and positive experience.

## The case study

These two images led us to mount a case study of a source of more routine images of care work with older people. We selected a popular weekly magazine: (a) because it has a wide circulation among welfare workers in the UK; (b) because it is distributed free to many agencies that employ and train them (in 1994 the audited readership was 262,000[1]); and (c) because, through its use of illustrations, it contributes directly to the popular image of care work. The magazine is directed specifically to those involved in social care as opposed to nursing or medical care. It contains an editorial comment section, news items and feature articles relating to policy and practice, and is an important source of job advertisements in the field of social work and social care. It is unlikely that the 262,000 actually read the magazine, from cover to cover. Nevertheless, it is probable that, even in the act of flicking through the pages, the conjunction of headlines and photographic illustration has an impact – regardless of whether or not the article is read (Hunter 1987; Johnson 1993). As has been proved by the success of commercial advertising, the repetition of image and message is absorbed and has cumulative effects upon subsequent attitudes and behaviour.

We included in our database all editions of this magazine from November 1978 to June 1994. From this, we selected out all photographic illustrations which met the following criteria: (a) they featured an older person and a younger person; and (b) they were directly linked to an article – not an advertisement – concerning paid care. These criteria presented us with occasional problems in determining who was an older person and what constituted paid care. When faced with uncertainty, we adopted the principle of 'if in doubt, include'. This trawl generated a sample of 328 illustrations. These included 270 different images. A total of 58 were duplicates – the same photograph was used to illustrate different articles.

## The content of the photographs

We initially organized the 270 photographs into four overlapping categories:

1 There are 47 photographs that we classified as 'teacher shots'. In these the younger person is portrayed as showing the older person or persons how to do something, is supervising them doing something or helping them to understand something. Often there are several older people who are sitting while the younger person stands or sits on a raised seat. Their positions and postures imply a teacher–pupil or supervisor–supervisee relationship, and the elevated position of the worker suggests an element of control in this relationship. Although these images frequently present a care relationship in that the younger person's attention is directed at one particular older person, the presence of other people indicates that this kind of interaction is shared. Older people are often cared for in groups.

2 There are 61 examples of 'portrait snapshots'. Here the participants are unambiguously posing for the camera, smiling as if the photograph was intended for the family album. As Patricia Holland (1991: 4) comments in her writing about family snapshots, 'There is no attempt to conceal the process of picture-taking – participants present themselves directly to the camera in an act of celebratory cooperation.' Many of these photographs are designed to demonstrate a bond of affection – touch, arms round shoulders, hugs etc. The nature of the caring relationship is portrayed primarily in familial terms, often, for example, as if the two were mother and daughter. Again, the worker in these shots tends to be in an elevated position – sitting on the arm of the chair, with his or her arm round the older person – implying that caring involves an element of control.

3 The third category includes 113 'caring for' shots. The younger person now is seeing to the physical needs of the older person, undertaking some task that helps the older person with daily living: cleaning the house, escorting, buttoning up a cardigan, feeding or seeing to feet. These photographs present the image of tending: that aspect of care that is concerned with physical needs (Parker 1981). They also present images of dependency, of older people who have to rely on others for practical help. In some instances, they present an image of senility, and it is primarily in these photographs that there are older people who show no sign of being aware of the camera. In contrast, some of these photographs are taken on the doorstep: the younger person delivering a meal or, clipboard in hand, undertaking some kind of assessment. The older person controlling the front door provides an image of supported or assisted independence rather than dependency.

4 Finally, the most common care image is that of the 144 'caring about' shots. This fourth type does not involve any physical assistance or supervisory work. Often the photograph does not include anyone other than the carer and the cared-for, both seemingly unaware of the camera's presence. It is a purely caring about relationship that is portrayed. Through hand-holding and eye-to-eye contact, an image of mutual concern is conveyed. A few (11 in total) of these photographs are of named politicians or local dignitaries visiting and 'caring about' an older person.

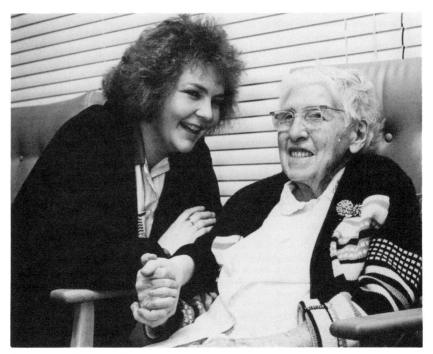

*An example of a 'caring about' image*
Photograph: John Birdsall

Analysing these 144 'caring about' images in a little more detail reveals something of the character of this dominant image. In the large majority of cases both 'carer' and 'cared about' are women (79 per cent of the younger persons and 87 per cent of the older persons). In the majority of instances, the younger person is looking at the older person (59 per cent). Often the older person is reciprocating (44 per cent) but sometimes he or she is looking towards the camera (19 per cent), at some object (15 per cent) or nowhere in particular – it would appear – (22 per cent). Frequently they are smiling (48 and 40 per cent of younger and older persons respectively). Occasionally they are touching: in 30 per cent of the photographs the younger person is touching the older person's hand, shoulder or occasionally arm or leg. In 19 per cent of the photographs they are touching a shared object: a cup of tea being the most common.

There is a marked difference in their positions. Most often the older person is sitting in a chair (69 per cent), sometimes standing (20 per cent) and occasionally in bed or in a wheelchair. In contrast the younger person is typically standing (49 per cent) or sitting in a chair (38 per cent). Less often they are in a kneeling position beside the older person's chair (10 per cent). In a majority of photographs, the younger person is leaning towards the older person (55 per cent) and occupies more space in the picture than the latter (57 per cent).

These statistics convey an image that is in part symmetrical – two women, looking at each other and smiling. In some there appears to be a conscious effort on the part of the younger person through kneeling or crouching to face the older person at the same level. In part, however, the image is also asymmetrical – the younger woman more often standing, touching, leaning and being more prominent in the picture. Often the older person appears as an 'exhibit', since the younger person, like the viewer, seems to be 'inspecting' her. Often there is an element of patronizing admiration. In the few photographs that feature young men as care workers, there is an air of jollity and informality, with the older women smiling or laughing.

On the matter of touch, it is often difficult to interpret how this comes about. Often it results from the younger person supporting the older, or helping her to her feet. Often it appears symmetrical: a mutual holding of hands. But in other instances, the position of the hands and the inclination of the bodies suggests that it is the younger person who has reached out. This suggests a conscious effort to include touch in the image of care that is being presented. In some pictures, where there is no touch, there is an inclination of one or both towards the other, which seems to be a gesture of warmth of feeling, of closeness in the relationship.

## The changing concept of care

The above analysis confirms that these four images of care-giving, and in particular the fourth 'caring about' image, have been dominant in the portrayal of care and older people over the past ten or twenty years.

It is interesting to compare them with the images included in Townsend (1962). Several of the captions to Townsend's photographs refer to 'the warden', 'the matron' and 'attendants'. There is no mention of 'care staff' or 'care assistants'. Indeed, the word 'care' does not appear in the index to the book. Compare this with more recent publications on residential care: for example, Willcocks et al. (1987) have 21 separate entries under 'care' in their index. Despite this, the concept of care was not unused in policy in the early post-war period: the National Assistance Act 1948, for example, placed a duty on local authorities to provide 'residential accommodation for persons . . . in need of care and attention'. Arguably, however, 'care and attention' is a different concept from what we now know of as care. We would speculate that care at the time of Townsend's research was still very much associated with hospital care – in many residential homes the staff were nurses and wore nurse uniforms. The notion of social care only took root in the 1970s after the creation of social services departments and the expansion of domiciliary services. The economic retrenchment and the shift towards community care which has characterized social policy since the mid-1970s has resulted in informal carers (unpaid family, neighbours and friends) being seen as an increasingly important resource, and this is reflected in a series of policy documents in the early 1980s. This interest in informal care led to a wealth of research into the subject of care and caring that has had a significant impact in turn on the paid care services.

The conclusion we draw is that the magazine has contributed to these historical changes by promoting an image of paid carers who 'care about' as well as 'care for' older people. However, rather than a symmetrical image of two people of different generations, each caring about the other (as is presented in the Counsel and Care photographs), the 'caring about' images that have been selected for publication in the magazine incorporate a view of older people as passive, controlled and dependent.

## The photographic illustrations in context

Since November 1988 the magazine has declared that: 'Unless stated all photographs are from library stock and the person or situations portrayed therein do not relate to the matters raised in the accompanying article.' This is a form of protection against litigation, as is the label 'posed by models', which is sometimes found beside a photograph. It is often the case that the photograph does indeed seem to be posed. When, however, the photograph is taken in what appears to be a group care setting, it seems probable that the older person *is* a user of that service and that the younger person *is* a care worker. It is when there is an imputation, perhaps implied by the accompanying article, that the people in the photograph have characteristics which they do not have in real life – having dementia or being a doctor, for example – that statements such as 'posed by models' protect the publisher.

The art editor may have no information about the origins of the photograph other than what is apparent from its content and title. Often the title is no more than a cryptic caption written on the back of the bromide, intended simply to distinguish it within a large collection of photographs. Thus a proportion of the photographs published by the magazine are not *commissioned* to illustrate particular points contained in particular articles. They are not documentary in the tradition established by magazines such as *Picture Post*. Of the 328 photographs we reviewed, only 86 (26 per cent) are of named persons or locations that feature in the reports or articles they accompany.

There are 62 examples of photographs which come from the same assignment but accompany unrelated articles in different editions. These are identifiable by the fact that they include the same person or persons wearing the same clothes, and are credited to the same photographer. Some of these series may be used over a considerable period of time. For example, five different photographs from the same assignment were published to accompany articles in different editions between 1982 and 1989.

Furthermore, in their repeat appearances, persons from the same assignment may be presented in very different guises, their identities being transformed through the use of new captions relating to very different articles. One young man, for example, first appears in a photograph accompanying an article on whistle-blowing published in July 1992. Here, he is described as a residential care worker. Two months later, he reappears with a client in her own home, in an article on the registration and inspection of domiciliary care agencies. And then, in January 1993, he appears again to illustrate an article on charging policies. In each photograph, he is wearing the same outfit – shorts, sweatshirt and trainers. Just before submitting this paper for publication, we noticed him again in an edition published in January 1995 accompanying an article on a hospital discharge scheme in Wales. The caption reads: 'In eight months joint working has delivered tangible results and other SSDs are watching the North Wales project with interest.' This last one is a good example of what Featherstone and Hepworth mean by 'immediacy and facticity', mentioned earlier. Not only are these real people in the photograph, but the belief that the young man is really a worker on a hospital discharge scheme is reinforced by the mention of time and location in the caption. The fact that the reader is informed that other SSDs are 'watching' the project adds further to the impression the young man is indeed working on discharge arrangements. Hence we can easily be forgiven for conflating image and reality.

As well as different photographs from the same assignment, we also found examples of the *same* photograph being used to illustrate different articles. A total of 38 photographs appeared twice in our sample and ten were used three times. One photograph, for example, of two women, the older in a chair and the younger leaning towards her, appeared in three different editions between May 1993 and April 1994. In all three editions, it is recorded that the photograph came from library stock and is posed by models. The three captions read:

1 Money matters: elderly people are often unaware of the choice they have if they are unexpectedly discharged into care.
2 Carers and clients can both be losers if local authorities fail to consider all the relevant factors, not just cost.
3 A Department of Health initiative aims to encourage developments in day and domiciliary care, and involves 15 local authorities.

In the second, the younger woman is clearly cast as an informal carer. The right-hand margin cuts out what is apparent from her first and third appearance – that she is in fact wearing a nurse's uniform. We also noticed that the area behind the nurse appears to have been blanked out. In the original, another person or persons may have been present. Whatever the case, the photograph appears to have been edited in order to represent the essence of the one-to-one care relationship. There are 12 other examples which appear to be based on this kind of detailed editing.

Through repetition, these duplicates become particularly memorable images of care work with older people. A number of them may be staged using models dressed for the part. The effect of this, in our view, is often to caricature the stereotype of the care relationship.

## Conclusion

The concept of care is central to the magazine we studied, and photographic illustrations are crucially important in immediately conveying what care means and how it is given. The analysis provides evidence that the majority of the illustrations are not simply documentary but are taken from library stock in order to promote specific images of care, images which can be recognized by the readership as reflecting their experience of care-giving. We know little about the origin of these library photographs. It seems probable that most were taken in order to meet the demands of the market.

The *Freelance Photographer's Market Handbook* assists the photographer by indexing subjects and by identifying magazines interested in each 'type of picture' (Tracy and Gibson 1992: 12). It emphasizes the need to offer images that are both familiar and different:

> Editors see a lot of pictures every day. The vast majority are totally unsuited to their market. Of those that are suited, many are still rejected because, despite being the right *type* of pictures, the subjects are still uninspiring. They are subjects the editor has seen over and over again; and the type that he [*sic*] will already have on file . . . If you want to make yours sell, you have to show that editor something different.
>
> (Tracy and Gibson 1992: 15–16)

This quote indicates the extent to which an organized market has developed in the UK in the production and distribution of illustrative photographs. As is the case with libraries of books, the promotion of 'efficient trading' has led to the development of commercial libraries with keyworded data banks relating to 'types of pictures'.

Beloff draws attention to the 'rules of the pose', which 'must allow us to show ourselves in some socially *correct* manner' (Beloff 1985: 211, our emphasis). The smile, for example, can be the classic cover up. So what these photographs tell us about care and older people is limited. But they tell us a good deal about the cultural construction of valued images among various professional groups. It is clear that the magazine has been attempting to strike a balance between the image of older people as dependent and in need of care and control and the image of a mutual caring relationship.

There is a considerable literature on the political implications of photographic images associated with disability (Barnes 1992; Hevey 1992; Shakespeare 1994). Familiar images for representing disability are being critically examined and a new approach is being developed. Central to this are two issues: the representation of care and dependence (Oliver 1990; Morris 1991), and the roles of photographer and viewer. This is summarized in the following comment from a review of the exhibition 'A Sense of Self':

> The exhibition as a whole is not a continuation of those 1970s projects of so-called 'positive images', but an attempt to reinvent the visualisation of personal experience of disability. The photographs reject the notion of heroic and angelic 'independence' which is little more than pressure to deny one's needs and not to be a nuisance to anybody . . . The project as a whole is a powerful piece because . . . through devices of identification such as direct address to camera, camera angle, and often the use of quizzical expressions, [it] manages to create an intimate complicity between the subject and the viewer.
>
> (Evans 1989: 51–2)

There is a wealth of photographic images of later life which are a world apart from those we find in magazines such as the one we have studied. There are many photographers, such as Cotier, Cunningham and Abrahams,[2] who have created realistic and challenging images of later life and who have ignored the association between age, care and dependence. What is lacking, it would appear, is a demand from the market for such images in the welfare and later life literature.

## Acknowledgement

We would like to thank Mike Hepworth and Andrew Blaikie for their comments on an earlier draft of this chapter.

## Notes

1  Personal communication.
2  James Cotier produced a collection of nude photographic portraits of older men and women in his book *Nudes in Budapest* (London: Aktok, 1991). Imogen Cunningham's photographs of old age were produced, when she was in her nineties, for her third book *After Ninety*, which was first published in 1977 by University of Washington Press, Seattle and London. Mike Abrahams produced all the photographs that were published in Gladys Elder's challenging book *The Alienated: Growing Old Today* (London: Writers and Readers Publishing Co-operative, 1977). Many of these photographs were reproduced in the Open University's course 'An Ageing Population', 1979.

## References

Barnes, C. (1992) *Disabling Imagery and the Media* (for the British Council of Organisations of Disabled People). Halifax: Ryburn Publishing.
Beloff, H. (1985) *Camera Culture*. Oxford: Basil Blackwell.
Blaikie, A. (1994) Photographic memory, ageing and the life course, *Ageing and Society*, 14(4), 479–97.
Counsel and Care (1993) *News: Advice and Help for Older People*, Autumn/Winter.
Counsel and Care (1994) *News: Advice and Help for Older People*, Spring/Summer.
Evans, J. (1989) A Sense of Self, *Ten 8*, 31, 50–2.
Evers, H. (1983) Elderly women and disadvantage: perceptions of daily and support relationships, in D. Jerrome (ed.) *Ageing in Modern Society*. London: Croom Helm.
Featherstone, M. and Hepworth, M. (1993) Images of ageing, in J. Bond, P. Coleman and S. Peace (eds) *Ageing in Society*, 2nd edn. London: Sage.
Gearing, B. and Slater, R. (1979) Images and perspectives, in *An Ageing Population P252*, Unit 2. Milton Keynes: The Open University.
Hevey, D. (1992) *The Creatures Time Forgot: Photography and Disability Imagery*. London: Routledge.
Holland, P. (1991) History, memory and the family album, in J. Spence and P. Holland (eds) *Family Snaps: the Meanings of Domestic Photography*. London: Virago.
Hunter, J. (1987) *Image and Word: the Interaction of Twentieth-century Photographs and Texts*. Cambridge, MA: Harvard University Press.
Johnson, M.K. (1993) (Re)framing the photograph, *Word and Image*, 9(3), 245–51.
Morris, J. (1991) *Pride Against Prejudice: Transforming Attitudes to Disability*. London: The Women's Press.

Oliver, M. (1990) *The Politics of Disablement*. Basingstoke: Macmillan.
Parker, R. (1981) Tending and social policy, in E.M. Goldberg and S. Hatch (eds) *A New Look at the Personal Social Services*. London: Policy Studies Institute.
Shakespeare, T. (1994) Cultural representation of disabled people: dustbins for disavowal?, *Disability and Society*, 9(3), 283–99.
Townsend, P. (1962) *The Last Refuge*. London: Routledge and Kegan Paul.
Tracy, J. and Gibson, S. (eds) (1992) *The Freelance Photographer's Market Handbook 1992*. London: BFP Books.
Willcocks, D., Peace, S. and Kellaher, L. (1987) *Private Lives in Public Places*. London: Tavistock.

## 12 JOANNA LATIMER

# Figuring identities: older people, medicine and time

## Prologue

> It is taken as quite natural that old age is a time of biological decline, which results in the entire population of older people being characterised by ill-health and sickness. To be old is to be unhealthy.
>
> (Victor 1991: 2)

> Take Jessie. She came to us as a purely social admission. She'd fallen at home and is incontinent. She had turned against her home help, refused to answer the door to let her in. She didn't become ninety-one over night, she's been old for a long time. She had been going downhill. She's been here ever since. She didn't have any medical problems.
>
> (A ward sister, acute medicine, field notes, Latimer 1994)

This chapter's starting place is the absurdity, yet the inescapability, of the category 'older people'. Older people are being treated as *a group*. The question addressed in the following discussion concerns the conditions under which the category 'older people' reappears, time after time. The position offered is not a comfortable one: it is not content with pointing the finger to suggest a conspiracy theory over why older people are downgraded and marginalized. Rather, the presumption is that almost all of us are implicated, even if it is only through fear of our own ageing, associated with loss rather than gain, physical decline rather than spiritual attainment, entrapment rather than liberation, and the death that these forebodings harbinger.

In the first passage quoted above the author points to a stability: in a British context, illness in old age is taken for granted as a 'natural' consequence of *biological decline*. The second passage points to how this assumption is not just taken for granted, to inform one practitioner's view of older people. It is being *deployed* by her. It is helping her to accomplish Jessie's disposal. Not from hospital, because at the current time there is nowhere for Jessie to go, but *partially*, from Sister's sense of responsibility for her.

Where an older person's difficulties can be explained, like Jessie's, as the effects of going downhill over time, their 'position', in an acute medical unit at least, can be diminished. In Sister's account, for example, it appears that Jessie's difficulties are the effects of *becoming* 91. Jessie's illness, or at least the effects she displays, is being constituted as the natural consequence of getting older, of decline. This infers, and plays upon, a difference: a distinction between illness effects which are the consequence of ageing, and other illness effects. It could be asked, 'Well, when are illness effects not "natural", when are they ever outside of nature?' It is this very interface which is of interest here, the interface between illness which must be accepted as part of life's course, and other kinds of illness, between natural and unnatural illnesses.[1]

Under particular conditions, illness framed as the inevitable consequence of biological time enables a shift in responsibility from medical practitioners, like Sister, and there can be a deferral. Jessie can be left off Sister's busy agenda. However, how Jessie's needs are being constituted are matters of interpretation. We need not think of these interpretations as only technical. Sister is giving an 'account', which is doing important ordering work.

Jessie, for example, has had a massive stroke, which would usually imply the presence of pathology, and a 'medical condition', but Sister absents this aspect of Jessie's situation from her account. And it is this absence that makes Sister's account so interesting. In absenting Jessie's stroke she is able to return Jessie to person, to *old* person, to someone whose illness is outside the domain of the medical ward of which she is in charge. Sister enrols the calendar of the years, Jessie's unsociable and unreasonable behaviour (perhaps hinting at dementia), her falls and her incontinence, to figure Jessie *as* an old person, rather than an acutely ill person. And notice, there is not just the degeneration of the body being implied, but of the mind as well: Jessie is irrational. She is being 'figured' almost as an un-person and, critically, she is being constituted as partly to blame, she has put herself beyond the pale. The listeners (myself, some of the staff nurses) are being given an account.

Through this account we are being 'moved': we may have seen Jessie in various ways, as an object of our concern and duty, but Sister is refiguring Jessie for us. Sister is unintentionally (or not) 'priming' us. Jessie is being put 'outside' one division, a class of patient (the person who is acutely ill), and into another class (that of old person whose difficulties are chronic and the consequence of a natural order of things, a progressive deterioration and decline).

I will argue that, rather than simply thinking of Sister as lying or as incompetent, we can think of her differently. Sister is both drawing on and reproducing an ambivalence to figure Jessie's identity and categorize her as 'old'. She is persuading us, and herself, perhaps, that Jessie is out of place, in every sense. For Jessie, the future is being presented as a continued slow and relentless decline to death: there is to be no possibility of a heroic story of recovery; for Sister, Jessie is a 'blocked bed'.

My suggestion, then, is that research on ageing should take the enigma of 'grouping' seriously, but as 'lived categories'. A lived category is produced through countless artefacts and occasions: through, for example, ceremonial moments in the life course like retirement or birthdays, the death of friends and partners, media and other literary and pictorial representations of older people, cashing in the pension book and, of concern in the current chapter, medical discourses and the older person's encounters with health care professionals (Cohen 1994; Kaufman 1994). These artefacts and occasions may include representations of older people which insist on stereotypical images, such as the road sign where a silhouette of a bent couple, the man brandishing a walking-stick, warns of the possible presence of older pedestrians; or the systematic exclusion of older people, for example, from television or cinema productions. These presences and absences help to tell each of us, not just the social and anthropological researcher, a great deal about how older people and old age are constituted in a society. Indeed, they help to circulate and reproduce the ways in which older people are constituted by themselves and by others in day-to-day life.

The rest of the chapter discusses one approach to studying the practices of people like doctors and nurses as they go about their everyday ordering work, and as they explain and give accounts of their work, to explicate some of the conditions of possibility under which 'older people' as a lived category is produced and reproduced.

## Introduction to the approach

The diversity and heterogeneity of older people and the danger of lumping older people together as a category are taken as read. As Featherstone and Hepworth (1991) have emphasized, the experience of old age as a category is partially a mask, a socially, economically and culturally constructed one. Behind the mask lies difference. However, rather than ending there, and saying that there is no such thing as 'older people', that it is only a story of stereotypes, we will accept 'older people' as a lived category.

If we accept that 'older people' is a lived category a critical question edges into view. This question is an anthropological one and concerns how it is that older people are continuously lumped together. It is not just that people of a certain age are considered together. Older people are lumped together in ways which have distinct political and personal consequences, in ways which, it must be emphasized, are both advantageous and disadvantageous to older people themselves (see, for example, Minkler 1995). There is then a distinct focus to the present chapter, suggested by the work of Latour (1986, 1987) and other contemporary social theorists (Strathern 1991, 1992a, 1993): rather than treat stable categories or social identities, such as 'older people', as the taken for granted effects of discourse, prejudice or stereotyping, passed on and diffused through society, it is the very appearance and reappearance of such a stable effect which requires explanation.

The approach discussed in the current chapter focuses on the distinctions which professional carers put into play to figure the identities of people like Jessie, as one of the locations through which old age and older people get reproduced as a cultural category. These distinctions can be considered as 'givens', as matters of expert interpretation, simply requiring the objective, experienced and informed gaze of the good nurse, doctor and social worker, the multidisciplinary team favoured by geriatricians and others concerned with the health and welfare of older people. The difficulty would then be whose view of the patient must be believed to be the true version.

Along with other sociological and anthropological studies of medical practices (Buckholdt and Gubrium 1979; Silverman 1987; Berg 1992; Becker and Kaufman 1995), the position taken in the current approach is that there is far more at stake to how health professionals make their distinctions and categorize people as patients for treatment and care. In this view, professionals are considered as members of societies, organizations and institutions. But membership is not simply conferred, it has to be worked at, or 'performed'.

A common view of encounters and interactions is to limit interpretation of what occurs to matters of individual interest. Here, within encounters, 'each person adopts a number of positions in which he or she expresses a sense of self, attempts to exert control over others, attempts to construct meaning' (Ritter 1995: vii). Self is something fixed, and the moves people make involve individuals.

Following an ethnomethodological tradition, encounters between persons can be viewed differently. They are occasioned or situated (Silverman 1993). Participants do not have selves, which they can or cannot present; they are performing within institutional and cultural orders. And critically, such performances help to reproduce institutional and cultural orders. In this view, then, individuals are subjects, but their subjectivities are not taken to be the products of individual choice, motivation, prejudice, ignorance or intention, but are 'constituted in specific institutional and discursive practices' (Silverman 1987: 134). Participants are not performing 'self' as individual (although it may be very important to give the appearance that this is what is being done). Instead, 'self' is seen as constituted through participation as member. Through their everyday conduct the participants perform their membership. In other words, the activities of nurses and doctors, especially those activities concerned with diagnosing and treating patients, can be considered as more than *a function* of the organization or the institution in which they work. Such activities can be construed as helping a performance of self as member and, through this, as helping to produce and reproduce that organization (Bittner 1973), society *and* a moral order (Garfinkel 1967; Silverman 1993).

For performance to be persuasive of membership, physical activities alone will rarely do. Members' accounts must make what participants do visible, as rational or as having rationale. That is, only some accounts will do: what 'counts' is itself situated. Getting to know what will serve as an account is all part of 'doing' (Garfinkel 1967) nurse, doctor or, for that matter, patient.

## Field work: the method

The acute medical unit[2] which formed the setting for the current ethnography consisted of one male and one female ward (wards 1 and 2) in a large and prestigious British hospital. Between the two wards there were 58 beds.

Field work included systematic collection of research material. Methods consisted of participant observation, interviews with nurses and patients, and transcription of all inpatient medical and nursing records. Specific locations observed included all aspects of patient management, as follows:

- the patient's admission, including the medical and nursing history and examination;
- observation of patients for regular two-hour periods throughout their stay in hospital;
- the geriatrician's assessment;
- home assessment visits where arranged (with the occupational therapist, social workers and community nurses);
- nurses' change of shifts reports;
- doctors' ward rounds;
- the social round or geriatric ward round – a type of multidisciplinary case conference.

All talk and actions in the encounters observed were recorded *verbatim* using a shorthand notation. These shorthand notes were transcribed within the same day on to a computer. In this way the research material consisted as far as possible of the words and actions of those in the setting, rather than the researcher's recall of those words, which would inevitably result in even more mediation.

Field notes were organized into chronological texts for each patient. In addition, field notes were also made on the ways in which each ward was organized, both internally (for example, the ways in which space was organized, how work was allocated and timed, staffing levels, skill mix, visiting times) and in relation to the overall organization of the hospital (e.g. how the ward was 'on take' for acute admissions). All aspects of hospital life, technical or otherwise, were taken as artefacts, as, like anything else we make, having the potential to be invested with meaning and to 'move participants' to position them. In this respect I made notes as to how each ward felt and about things which struck me about the way they were. I also spent a lot of time with people, with nurses and patients particularly, but also in conversation with doctors, physiotherapists, families and others. Informal occasions like these provided impressions and materials for helping to explain why things worked in the ways they did in the setting.

For example, while striding down the corridor with a senior consultant, met by chance on his way to his office, I had a conversation which much later helped me to 'see' something about the ways in which doctors and nurses performed. The doctor was talking to me about the archaic structure of the building and in passing he said that they (this unit, the staff) were trying to accomplish 'the provision of first class medicine in a Third World environment'. The idea of 'first class medicine' resonated on and on through many performances and accounts, those of both nurses and doctors. It was one of the repertoires available: they were there not just to provide first class medicine, but to *do* it, to keep it going through their performances as one of the great British institutions, one of the heroic projects of modernity. But, as we have already seen with Jessie, what constitutes medicine is a movable feast; having a stroke doesn't necessarily make you medical. To practise first class medicine, you have to have first class patients. And the managerial conditions which facilitate this entail turnover. To focus on a first class patient means others have to be turned over, faster and faster.

One of the most important artefacts which health care professionals have available to them to produce their performances is the identity of the patient. By identity here I mean particularly how a person is identified *as* a patient, in other words his or her medical and non-medical identity, to use the distinction which practitioners, such as Sister quoted above, themselves use. Sister stated that Jessie was a 'purely social admission', she had no 'medical' problems. The identities of professionals can be understood to be integrated with the identities of the patients they treat. These artefacts, patients' identities, are constructed on many occasions and through diverse practices: on ward rounds, through medical records, nurses' reports, at the bedside, to name but a few. However, this is not to suggest that professionals can assemble *any* identity for their patients: the availability of materials and devices through which to figure the identity of patients is contextually situated, there is a *logic* to the context which participants produce and reproduce. And, critically, as seen in the case of Jessie, professionals may also be as concerned to disassemble the identities of people *as* patients, to enable their disposal.

In order to research how the identities of older people are constituted through the practices of doctors and nurses, an ethnographic research method is the method of choice, as it allows examination of the specific discursive and institutional practices through which identities are constituted. The methods should provide enough detail for a theoretical analysis which can (tentatively and provisionally) explain (Latour 1991; Silverman 1993) the reasons why people are conducting themselves in particular ways rather than others. Central to this position is the notion that participants, doctors and nurses in the current setting, are accomplishing particular forms of identity and organization (Garfinkel 1967; Bittner 1973). But they are not organizing just one domain, but many (Strathern 1992a). As Silverman's (1987) study of a diabetic clinic suggests, in organizing treatment and care for young diabetics, the doctors, parents and patients are also organizing cultural and social mores to do with responsibility and autonomy, parenting and family, youth and adulthood. So family, as a cultural form, is organized not just through family life, but also in such places as the clinic. Similarly, old age and older people as a cultural category are organized through many practices, including those which help to organize the current hospital setting.

The specific analytic methods developed involved textual analysis[3] of each set of research material for one ward. Interpretations were then cross-checked with material collected on the other ward. A critical analytic approach was developed, which drew on both anthropology and discourse analysis (Silverman 1987, 1993). The texts compiled from the accounts (written, verbal, to each other, to the researcher, formal and informal) of those in the setting were analysed in relation to both their forms, as *devices*, and their content, as *materials*. As devices and materials (Czarniawska–Joerges 1997), the accounts have been critically examined for what they make present and what they make absent, for the identities and social relations they constitute and which constitute them.

The scale was consistently changed (Strathern 1991) through examining the discourses and practices of participants in relation to one patient and then comparing this with other patients, other participants and the other ward. Rather than seeing information as 'falsifiable' (Popper 1969) it was interpreted to reveal differences or tensions between cases or situations. Further, different discursive events were compared for form and content: for example, the ward round as compared with a nursing change of shift report or a nurse–patient interview.

## Geriatric assessment: producing and reproducing categories

To illustrate the approach, one particular finding will be presented, drawing on a detailed example. From the analysis, the purpose of the 'social round' is to discuss the older patients in relation to their medical diagnosis and treatments, their rehabilitation and their social situation, but mainly in respect of how any of these may impede their discharge. The way in which the social round was managed appeared to be quite explicitly aimed at bringing to light actual or potential impediments to a patient's discharge, and to ensure that all possible care is taken to mobilize resources to enable as speedy and safe a discharge as possible, in whatever form this might take. The round can be considered as a form of audit to check that staff are doing their work thoroughly and well in relation to getting patients through.

The first extract comes from the occasion of the social round, or multi-disciplinary ward meeting, at which all the patients over the age of 65 were discussed.[4] Here there is a presentation of a patient which contrasts well with the example of Jessie cited above.

> Present at the meeting are: consultant geriatrician, two staff nurses (wards 1 and 2), two physiotherapists, social worker, medical student, speech therapist, researcher, two residents who come in after meeting has started.
>
> *Consultant geriatrician*: Bernard Gibbon is a 76-year-old man who came in having collapsed with hypotension, he's got known arterial disease[?]. He lives with his wife who attends the day hospital at Southmount. Home help five times a week, meals on wheels three days a week. So they're obviously a problem.[5] [Looks up at staff nurse.]
> *Staff nurse*: His wife – she's not able to see, so I don't think she does much.
> *Consultant geriatrician*: Does he do anything for her?
> *Staff nurse*: I don't think so.
> *Consultant geriatrician*: So they just coexist – with community support.
>
> 1 min 4 seconds

Mr Gibbon is figured by the geriatrician as a patient who, in conjunction with his wife, is 'obviously a problem'. The 'problem' is signalled by a number of factors: the patient has long-term disabling illness (arterial disease); his wife attends a day hospital which signifies she has physical/emotional disability; and they are already reliant on home help to maximum frequency, as well as meals on wheels.

The consultant checks whether Mr Gibbon does anything for his wife, the staff nurse thinks not, and the consultant makes the statement that they 'just coexist – with community support'. At this point staff have not identified any particular impediments to discharge, and go no further. Mr Gibbon is being figured as medical and as having social problems associated mainly with his wife.

Subsequently, Mr Gibbon is reported on at the nurses' ward reports as 'difficult to mobilize'. This becomes an issue: he is described as always lying in bed, apparently reluctant to get up, to wash and 'be independent'. Here is the discussion at the intermediate social round. Mr Gibbon has been in for ten days at this point:

> Present at the meeting are: senior registrar for geriatrics, occupational therapist, two physiotherapists, two staff nurses (wards 1 and 2), social worker, resident (ward 2), medical student, researcher.
>
> *Senior registrar* (geriatrics): Bernard Gibbon, an arteriopath. Collapsed with horrendous hypotension [low blood pressure].
> *Resident*: He has paroxysmal AF [atrial fibrillation, a heart arrhythmia] on ECG [electrocardiogram], so he's started on digoxin [a drug which slows and regulates the heart beat]. He feels very tired – I can't find any reason for it – his Us and Es [urea and electrolytes] are normal, he's not constipated, no UTI [urinary tract infection], his spit is negative. I cannot think why he's so tired except that he's lying in bed all the time. We keep trying to get him up – the nurses keep trying to get him up but . . .
> *Senior registrar* (geriatrics): Is he depressed?[6]
> *Resident*: No! He's really cheerful. Whenever I speak to him it's 'Aye doctor, yes doctor' [robustly] then . . . [Resident throws his head back and snores loudly]!! [Everyone laughs. Senior registrar smiles but does not laugh.]
> *Social worker*: He's a bit like you then [the resident has been asleep earlier in the meeting]! [Laughs, everyone laughs.]
> *Resident*: And I'm not constipated either. [Laughs.]
> *Senior registrar* (geriatrics): [he's stopped laughing] Has anybody asked him about that? [serious]
> *Resident*: No.
> *Senior registrar* (geriatrics): I got the impression things are pretty hefty at home – with his wife and all.
> *Resident*: She's in and out – she's psychotic I think.
> *Senior registrar* (geriatrics): She goes to the day hospital doesn't she?
> *Resident*: Yes – but there is some psychiatric history.
> *Senior registrar* (geriatrics): She may be demented.
> *Resident*: No – she's a very dependent personality – that's it. Also she's a cancer phobic.
> *Senior registrar* (geriatrics): Right, OK, he's really a medical problem – the home help five days a week is more for his wife than for him.

2 minutes

The resident begins by figuring Mr Gibbon as having medical problems. These are, however, easily definable as the effects of old age (a failing heart, arterial problems etc.). He goes on to suggest that Mr Gibbon is lying in bed all the time and that this is why he feels tired – he can find no pathological cause for his behaviour. The geriatrician (the senior registrar) calls the resident to account: there is an implicit charge (Silverman 1987, 1993) in his questioning of the resident as to whether the patient is depressed. The way the humour works here is interesting, as it could signify that the resident is actually embarrassed at some level at being put in this position. The resident claims that the patient is not depressed and accounts for this by a description of his behaviour. The geriatrician to some extent refuses the play acting and the jokes, and asks if anyone has talked to the patient about 'that' (presumably the question of Mr Gibbon's mood). The resident says no, he has not. The geriatrician accounts for his insistence by reference to the patient's so-called social history: 'I got the impression things are pretty hefty at home – with his wife and all.' The resident then covers himself a little by revealing that he has gone into the question of the wife in some detail, and knows she is a cancer phobic. This expression of knowledge about the patient's wife distracts from the revelation that he has not talked to the patient about how he feels. Then there is an odd turn: the geriatrician states that the home services are not really for the patient, who is a 'medical problem'. In returning Mr Gibbon to the medical, he suspends any further talk about Mr Gibbon's depression or his social problems, or indeed the problem of what has now been subtly constituted as his *reluctance* to mobilize. But the alert has been given: that the patient may not get going.

A few days later, the senior house officer interprets a routine chest X-ray to diagnose that Mr Gibbon has had a pneumonia for some time, and there is even some suspicion that he may have cancer. This accounts to the doctors for why the patient is so tired; they appear not too concerned to find out about how he feels, and they tell Mr Gibbon that they will send him home as soon as possible, so that he can go on looking after his wife. The patient begins to recover himself when he is moved to the side ward and is put on antibiotic medication and a nightcap to help him sleep. Mr Gibbon's 'hefty situation' is not explored, as far as I know.

In his interviews with me, both formal and informal, Mr Gibbon revealed his utter bleakness in relation to his future. For him his life at home was 'hell'. His wife had been made partially blind by a stroke. She had to 'feel her way' to get around. She did not do anything any more; he had to do everything in the house which the home help did not do. He said he could no longer get out of the house: could no longer walk any distance because his breath was so short. He said that he did not have any social life: they used to go to a club across the road several nights a week, but they no longer go because his wife cannot read the cards for bingo.

> *Mr Gibbon*: She doesn't go out so I don't go out either.
> *R*: So your social life now . . . ?
> *Mr Gibbon*: Is finished. I've no social life at all.

He told me his wife stopped him watching television, because she could not see it. Further, he could not sleep at night: he said he had been unable to sleep for months and months, but during the last few days of his stay he was able to sleep at night and felt less tired in the day.

He stated that what really got him down was that his wife never stopped complaining and going on to him. He felt that this was understandable and that she was terribly bitter about what had happened to her, but that he was trapped. Sometimes he said he had to go into another room 'to stop something from happening' (I assume he meant to stop himself from losing his temper or hitting her). During his interview with me he broke down and cried when talking about going home. This picture is a very different one from how he was being represented on the ward rounds. For him all his problems were inextricably linked together: the geriatrician had got it right when he said that he got the impression that things were pretty hefty at home.

In contrast to Jessie, Mr Gibbon is being returned to medical; the social support is more for his wife than for him. Does this merely indicate that the health care workers are insensitive, blind or incompetent in not being able to see Mr Gibbon's world as he sees it? Or are there critical moves here? Is there an alternative reading to what is going on?

## Accomplishing the flow

At first sight Mr Gibbon appears to have a medical identity, but that identity is marginal: his medical problems are after all mainly being constituted as owing to the problems of old age (he is an arteriopath, and there is not much that can be done about that). And staff have dealt with the medical problems as best they can: his blood pressure is under control, he has perked up and he is on some heart medicine. And, critically, he has been in for a long time. If Mr Gibbon were moved on to the social grounds as explanation for his observed behaviour, there is a risk that he may not get home: investigate his home situation too deeply while he is in hospital and they might be opening a can of worms. At this juncture holding him on medical grounds helps to keep him on the move.[7] And not even the most sympathetic geriatrician is keen to get involved with a blind old woman with possible dementia, cancer phobia and a personality disorder unless he has to. Perhaps staff are not being insensitive; perhaps they do in fact get a very good sense of just how difficult things could be for Mr Gibbon, but making them explicit may block their chances of getting him out.

While geriatric medical discourse as written appears as the ally of the aged, as it focuses attention not just on the older person's body, but on a more so-called holistic view, there are potential problems with such extensions. Underpinning the position of some geriatricians is the idea that illness in old age is not just the consequence of physical decline, a natural process, pathological, but that illness in old age is more complicated: illness in old age is connected to the other aspects of older people's lives, to their social situations, their ability to function and their psychological and emotional states. To accomplish a recentring of the person, practices are advocated which stress the imperative of early, formalized assessment and discharge planning, with strong functional and psycho-social components.

As both Silverman (1987) and Armstrong (1982) argue, these shifts in what is termed more social medicine, while encompassing many features recommended by medical reformers, also extend the range of medicine to practices and grounds which include the possibility for the subject to be constituted as other than a purely medical subject. In allowing what Armstrong (1982: 15) calls surveillance of 'the patient's environment and biography', these extensions make available methods for scrutinizing the resources accessible to the elderly person and compound associations between old age and the chronic and social dimensions of ill health, making available materials for a non-medical solution to the older person's problems to be arrived at. In the hands of participants, the access to a person's 'environment and biography' can mean that there are more available legitimate grounds upon which to figure a patient's identity.

What emerges in the current context is that an extension of assessment practices opens up the possibility for surveying for potential impediments to discharge early rather than late and, where potential impediments exist, grounds are available for shifting the identity of the patient to enable his or her disposal. While such distinctions help participants to manage the identities of both older people and themselves, in being deployed they are being recirculated, time and time again. And it is this latter point that is so important. In figuring the older person as patient, doctors and nurses are orchestrating distinctions, such as 'natural', 'social' and 'medical', with distinct political effects in terms of the local organizing work with which they are charged.

Geriatric assessment is just one of the things which is being 'translated' (Latour 1986) in the hands of participants to be reconfigured and, indeed, recomposed locally and specifically. Latour (1986: 267) explains translation as:

> the spread in time and space of anything – claims, orders, artefacts, goods – is in the hands of people; each of these people may act in many different ways, letting the token drop or modifying it, or deflecting it, to betraying it, or adding to it, or appropriating it.

The translations which occur are the effects of the particular configurations with which the participants are associated: the meanings interpreted for artefacts, the identities being constituted, the organizing being accomplished and the matters of interest involved. The translations are the effect of, and affect, particular sets of social relations. However, all translations which together produce and reproduce a consistent effect, such as the lumping together of older people as a cultural category, require examination and discussion. There has to be a *networking of interests* present for the appearance and reappearance of a stability to be maintained.

## Analytical attitude

The purpose of the current research enterprise has been to attempt to lay bare some of the networks of interest through which effects appear to be stabilized. The degree to which the ethnography can (tentatively and provisionally) represent the setting lies partly in the 'attitude' of the ethnographer in the analysis, towards his or her subjects.

An important aspect to the analytic attitude concerns 'judgement'. Judging participants' communicative practices as poor, as examples of 'bad communication' or 'bad practice', can be unhelpful. Giving up such judgements is difficult, but by viewing participants' practices as skilled (Silverman 1993) and by asking such questions as 'what might these practices be helping participants to accomplish', the ethnographer can try to grasp why participants conducted themselves in the ways they did.

What emerged in the current ethnography was something which appeared to be systematic: even where the strategies deployed differ, similar effects are accomplished over the ways in which the identities of patients *as* older are managed. The patients emerge throughout the research material as having ambivalent status, as potentially not authentic or inappropriate in some way, even where, like Jessie, there were quite clearly what would by any commonsense interpretation be termed 'medical' problems.

These effects are accomplished continuously, through a number of methods. These include a play and a tension over what constitutes 'illness', in particular the relationship between acute illness and other forms of illness, and what constitutes being 'naturally old' and therefore naturally ill. This effect is sometimes accomplished through a sequestration of patients' concerns and the effects they display, or, if these concerns are made present, methods for recategorizing them so that they can be deferred.

Over Jessie, for example, Sister, in the quote given at the beginning of the chapter, is playing on the notion that difficulties which are the consequence of a natural decline are not medical, they are social: she is classifying Jessie as being what Douglas (1989: 35) refers to as 'a matter out of place'. Jessie is representative of something which is *the matter* with Sister's ward. She is being constituted as someone who does not belong, she is not a medical problem, she is a geriatric, and this is a medical ward.

> R: So what is a 'geriatric' patient?
> *Sister*: Elderly.
> *Senior staff nurse*: Frail, old, gone off their legs a bit.
> (Field notes, Latimer 1994)

But alongside this categorizing was a continuous *grading* of categories of patient: some things were continuously worked to appear more important than others, so that 'problems' associated with the psycho-social were constantly downgraded, as less important than medical problems. Elsewhere I have discussed this extensively, drawing on the work of Bauman (1991), as the 'constituting of classes' (Latimer 1997). By associating the problems older people display with their age, or with their social situation, there is an immediate effect, a *downgrading* effect.

To understand the moves here it is critical to ask what staff are accomplishing. Rather than an assumption that they just have an attitude problem, that they are just stereotyping, what emerges is that they are making these distinctions in a particular organizational context of practice. Old age emerges as the grounds for explaining the effects a person displays in particular contexts. These include those patients whose 'illnesses' are not going away (like Jessie): reconstituting their 'problems' as owing to old age helps staff, like the nurses, to dispose of their responsibility towards the patients in the situation where these sorts of problems are of less importance than others.

So 'oldness', in whatever guise, may get deployed when someone cannot be moved: his or her problems are not medical, they are owing to 'old age'. This strategy allows for a deferral, a deferral and a justification. It also reproduces a cultural category: the old as naturally and inevitably ill. On other occasions the strategy may be very different, as with Mr Gibbon, but the effect similar: in contrast with Jessie, staff hold explanation for his troubles on clinical grounds, and he and his other concerns can be deferred.

## Concluding discussion

To accomplish their organizing work, participants move each other around, to get each other either to see what they are up to or to change the ways in which others see; in this way some encounters are either adversarial (Fernandez 1986) or agonistic (Lyotard 1983). To move and persuade participants draw on culturally available materials and devices (Strathern 1992b). As we have seen, they also underpin their positions with reasons and justifications, or what the ethnomethodologists call accounts. That is, their practices, both discursive and other, deploy organizing devices, and sets of materials which have to be persuasive to be performative. In these ways, through participants' performances which draw on materials that are already available, particular cultural and social entities get circulated and reproduced (see also Fernandez 1986). For example, that constipation, depression, chemical imbalance or infection as well as a person's 'social situation' can all cause depression in an older person are not accounts which are questioned in the social round concerning Mr Gibbon. These are all readily available repertoires. But what these repertoires do is also to make available different grounds upon which to explain the effects an older person displays. They put into play possibilities for figuring people as ill *because* they are old.

The findings of the current study suggest that in the hands of participants, in an acute medical setting at least, the associations and practices made available through geriatric assessment merged well with contemporary health care agendas driven by cost containment. Indeed, they seem to have helped to buttress strategies for increasing throughput within the acute sector. A further effect was continuously to narrow what constitutes the medical, to the exclusion of the social or the natural, and *thereby* to marginalize some older people, because, as we have seen, older people are systematically being associated with the natural and the social. Here there was a deferral of what perhaps the older person saw as his or her interests and concerns to other domains (for example, Mr Gibbon was *divided* from his wife, it was she not him who required the social care) or to the hands of other professionals. The effect of these practices of distinction was not simply the management of *patients'* identities. What is being suggested is that in the study of how doctors and nurses figure people's identities as patients (or not, as in the case of Jessie), what is being studied is the reproduction of cultural categories: both the identities of older people as a category which is distinguishable from other categories of people, and the identities of doctors and nurses who are, in this particular case, concerned primarily with not just any medicine, but first class, acute medicine.

Through the ways in which nurses and doctors figure older people as patients (or return the patient to person), they recursively reconstitute some of the very ways in which the identities of older people are categorized and the associations which 'old age' has in modernity. Geriatric assessment under certain conditions may make available the social and cultural construction of older people, and help to reproduce the very distinctions which it deploys.[8] This finding resonates with a statement of Hazan's: 'In the case of old age, information about the aged is used, wittingly or otherwise, to sustain the social position it reflects' (Hazan 1994: 2–3). But in the current case the concern has been to present a way of examining how old age and the identities of older people are constituted through the knowledge embedded in everyday practices.

Rather than reproducing what Silverman (1993: 22) calls a 'spurious' polarity between the natural, the social and the medical, the aim has been to see how these oppositions are played out in everyday life over the ways in which people are being figured as old in a medical context. And rather than critique the practitioners concerned for being ignorant or prejudiced, the study has examined what they are accomplishing through these communicative effects, namely the potential to shift identities and keep the appearance of the flow, the movement through the beds, the 'consultant episodes' which have since become one of the measures of efficiency and performance in the health services. None of this is to suggest that either the ward sisters or their colleagues felt comfortable about this situation. As I hope the chapter has indicated, to insist on judging these practitioners solely in such terms would be to forget that there are very complex practical, instrumental and existential reasons why someone such as Jessie was being figured the way she was. It would be to insist on returning practitioners to an odd group, the group of 'humans': persons whose notions of right and wrong exist before and above, perhaps even out of, everyday life. Rather than consider Sister as an individual, making decisions and choices, we can rethink her (and her nursing and medical colleagues) as *participant*. Through her conduct, Sister is performing to a wide and frequently conflicting set of criteria. She has not one simple identity, her self, to get across, but multiple identities to perform: as professional, with philosophies of caring to meet, as employee, as acute medical nurse, as manager, as citizen, to name but a few.

## Notes

1 It is the same ambivalence over the relationships between illness, age and nature which permits the query on hearing that someone's relation has recently died: 'How old was she?' When the bereaved replies that 'She was seventy-five', there has to be a judgement as to whether it is appropriate to offer the consolation that 'She has "had a good innings".' If the reply is that the deceased was fifty-five, then a different response might be in order, a gasp and a sympathetic look and the comment: 'My, that was young to have a stroke/heart attack/etc.' Under most conditions death at an even earlier age would begin to take on the proportions of the tragic.

2  I have argued extensively elsewhere how an acute medical unit in Britain can be considered a site of critical interest in relation to the constituting of the identities of older people (Latimer 1994). Alongside the health service as a target to be managed, emerges the critical case of ill older people. Indeed, I have wondered whether some of the impetus for reorganizing the health services in relation to social services has been an impulse partly constituted by the problem of older people. Towards the end of the 1970s 'older people' had become an explicit problem in relation to the acute sector. Debate carried on into the early 1980s (Alderson 1986; Bachman *et al.* 1987; Barker *et al.* 1985; Bouchier and Williamson 1982; Coid and Crome 1981; Hulter Asberg 1986) and continues today. Discussions link older people to time and ill-health in a way which is critical in relation to decisions over the distribution of resources.

3  Textual analysis was conducted as recommended by Fairclough (1992). It includes such things as taking account of the order and genre (narrative, interview, examination, conversation) of different types of discursive event. This was established through attention to such matters as how turn-taking and linguistic forms in interactions are operated by participants to maintain identities and establish hierarchies in social relations (see also Drew and Heritage 1992; Schegloff 1992; Heath 1992). For example, when analysing nurses' interviews with patients, I did not just pay attention to what was said but looked at how (or if) the interview was characterized by the nurse to the patient; who speaks and when; and how do they speak to each other, in a question and answer format or in a conversational format, or do they go in and out of different genres; is the format controlled and by whom; do they use jokes, when do they use jokes and what do they convey/communicate when they use jokes? Particular attention was paid to the language effects used, in particular to the place of particular forms of discourse (e.g. medical and nursing) and to metaphor and metonymy. Quantitative measures, such as the extent of a description and the time spent on its delivery, have also been taken into account.

4  In the present case, an acute medical unit, geriatrician consultation was a part of the management of older patients: all people over the age of sixty-five were assessed by a geriatrician and each week there was a multidisciplinary case conference in which each case was discussed. This conference was referred to as the 'social' round – once again associating illness in old age with the social, with matters beyond the scope of medicine. The emergence of the geriatric assessment is not just a local phenomenon: the inclusion of some form of geriatric assessment within the acute sector of the health services coincides with the rationalizing of the health services and is an aspect of the debates over older people mentioned above.

5  It emerged during field work that such matters as the presence and absence of relatives living at home and the frequency of visits by home help and other community workers acted as signs and could be read to indicate to ward staff how fragile the older person is at home. A high frequency of home visits is taken by them to indicate that the community support is already stretched to breaking point, without the added weight of any new, fresh illness and subsequent disability.

6  These as causes of Mr Gibbon's behaviour are all truisms in geriatric medical discourse: the patient may be sluggish and difficult to mobilize because he is depressed, constipated, has infection or electrolyte imbalance.

7  But the social grounds are being kept in play, they are there if need be: there are other cases in the study where the effects a person displays do not entirely go away and the patient is returned to person to enable a disposal (see Latimer 1997).

8  What Giddens (1984) and others have referred to as a process of 'recursion'.

## References

Alderson, M. (1986) An ageing population – some demographic and health trends, *Public Health*, 100, 263–77.

Armstrong, D. (1982) Medical knowledge and modalities of social control, mimeo. London: Unit of Sociology, Guy's Hospital Medical School.

Bachman, S., Collard, A., Greenberg, J., Fountain, E., Huebner, T., Kimbal, B. and Melendy, K. (1987) An innovative approach to geriatric acute care delivery: the Choate–Symmes experience, *Hospital and Health Services Administration*, 32(4), 509–20.

Barker, W.H., Williams, T.F., Zimmer, J.G., Van Buren, C., Vincent, S.J. and Pickrel, S.G. (1985) Geriatric consultation teams in acute hospitals: impact on back-up of elderly patients, *Journal of the American Geriatrics Society*, 33, 422–8.

Bauman, Z. (1991) The social manipulation of morality: moralising actors, adiaphorising action, *Theory, Culture and Society*, 8(1), 137–51.

Becker, G. and Kaufman, S.R. (1995) Managing an uncertain illness trajectory in old age: Patients' and physicians' views of stroke, *Medical Anthropology Quarterly*, 9(2), 165–87.

Berg, M. (1992) The construction of medical disposals. Medical sociology and medical problem-solving in clinical practice, *Sociology of Health and Illness*, 14(2), 151–80.

Bittner, E. (1973) The concept of organisation, in G. Salaman and K. Thompson (eds) *People and Organizations*. London: Longman/Open University Press.

Bouchier, I. and Williamson, J. (1982) The elderly patient in the acute hospital sector, *Health Bulletin*, 40(4), 179–82.

Buckholdt, D.R. and Gubrium, J.F. (1979) Doing staffings, *Human Organisation*, 38(3), 255–64.

Cohen, A. (1994) *Self-consciousness: an Alternative Anthropology of Identity*. London: Routledge.

Coid, J. and Crome, P. (1986) Bed blocking in Bromley, *British Medical Journal*, 292, 1253–6.

Czarniawska-Joerges, B. (1997) *Narrating the Organization: Dramas of Institutional Identity*. Chicago: Chicago University Press.

Douglas, M. (1989) *Purity and Danger. An Analysis of the Concepts of Pollution and Taboo*. New York: Ark Paperbacks.

Drew, P. and Heritage, J. (1992) Analysing talk at work: an introduction, in P. Drew and J. Heritage (eds) *Talk at Work. Interaction in Institutional Settings*. Cambridge: Cambridge University Press.

Fairclough, N. (1992) Discourse and text: linguistic and intertextual analysis within discourse analysis, *Discourse and Society*, 3(2), 193–217.

Featherstone, M. and Hepworth, M. (1991) The mask of ageing and the postmodern lifecourse, in M. Featherstone, M. Hepworth and B.S. Turner (eds) *The Body. Social Process and Cultural Theory*. London: Sage.

Fernandez, J.W. (1986) *Persuasions and Performances. The Play of Tropes in Culture*. Bloomington: Indiana University Press.

Garfinkel, H. (1967) *Studies in Ethnomethodology*. Englewood Cliffs, NJ: Prentice Hall.

Giddens, A. (1984) *The Constitution of Society. Outline of Structuration Theory*. Cambridge: Polity Press.

Hazan, H. (1994) *Old Age. Constructions and Deconstructions*. Cambridge: Cambridge University Press.

Heath, C. (1992) The delivery and reception of diagnosis in the general-practice consultation, in P. Drew and J. Heritage (eds) *Talk at Work*. Cambridge: Cambridge University Press.

Hulter Asberg, K.H. (1986) Elderly patients in acute medical wards and home care. Functional assessment, prediction of outcome, and a trial of early activation. PhD

Thesis, Comprehensive Summaries of Uppsala Dissertations from the Faculty of Medicine, 25, University of Uppsala, Sweden.

Kaufman, S.R. (1994) Old age, disease, and the discourse on risk: geriatric assessment in US health care, *Medical Anthropology Quarterly*, 8(4), 430–47.

Latimer, J. (1994) Writing patients, writing nursing: the social construction of nursing assessment of elderly patients in an acute medical unit. PhD thesis, University of Edinburgh.

Latimer, J. (1997) Giving patients a future: the constituting of classes in an acute medical unit, *Sociology of Health and Illness*, 19(2), 23–53.

Latour, B. (1986) The powers of association, in J. Law (ed.) *Power, Action and Belief: A New Sociology of Knowledge?* Sociological Review Monograph 32. London: Routledge and Kegan Paul.

Latour, B. (1987) *Science in Action*. Milton Keynes: Open University Press.

Latour, B. (1991) Technology is society made durable, in J. Law (ed.) *A Sociology of Monsters. Essays on Power, Technology and Domination*. London: Routledge.

Lyotard, J.F. (1983) *The Post-modern Condition: A Report on Knowledge*. Manchester: Manchester University Press.

Minkler, M. (1995) Critical perspectives on ageing: new challenges for gerontology. Opening Plenary, British Society of Gerontology Annual Conference, Keele University, England.

Popper, K. (1969) *Conjectures and Refutations*. London: Routledge and Kegan Paul.

Ritter, S. (1995) Foreword, in S. Tilley, *Negotiating Realities. Making Sense of Interaction between Patients Diagnosed as Neurotic and Nurses*. Aldershot: Avebury.

Schegloff, E.A. (1992) On talk and its institutional occasions, in P. Drew and J. Heritage (eds) *Talk at Work. Interaction in Institutional Settings*. Cambridge: Cambridge University Press.

Silverman, D. (1987) *Communication and Medical Practice. Social Relations in the Clinic*. London: Sage.

Silverman, D. (1993) *Interpreting Qualitative Data. Methods for Analysing Talk, Text and Interaction*. London: Sage.

Strathern, M. (1991) *Partial Connections*. Savage, MD: Rowman and Littlefield.

Strathern, M. (1992a) *After Nature. English Kinship in the Late Twentieth Century*. Cambridge: Cambridge University Press.

Strathern, M. (1992b) Writing societies, writing persons, *History of Human Sciences*, 5(1), 5–16.

Strathern, M. (1993) Society in drag, *Times Higher Educational Supplement*, 2 April, 19.

Victor, C.R. (1991) *Health and Health Care in Later Life*. Buckingham: Open University Press.

## 13 SARAH HARPER

# Constructing later life/constructing the body: some thoughts from feminist theory

## Introduction

As the feminist philosopher Grosz has recently pointed out, from its very foundation modern Western philosophy has faced a 'crisis of reason', which has taken many forms but remains essentially a conflict between objectivity and subjectivity. In her keynote article (1993) and subsequent text (1994) she sets out to explore the feminist challenge to the founding presumptions of Western rational thought, drawing out the implications of acknowledging the *body* in the production and evaluation of such knowledge.

> This crisis of reason is a consequence of the historical privileging of the purely conceptual or mental over the corporeal; that is, it is a consequence of the inability of Western knowledges to conceive their own processes of (material) production, processes that simultaneously rely on and disavow the role of the body.
>
> (Grosz 1993: 187)

In this chapter I wish to use Grosz's work on knowledge and the body as a frame within which to explore and attempt to understand the role of the ageing body in the social construction of later life. I shall argue that the ageing body remains pivotal to both our experience and construction of this process, and that this is primarily due to the manner in which the knowledge which defines the ageing body is itself produced and interpreted. In discussing this I shall draw on feminist theory regarding the sexed body and the production of sexed knowledge.

The following section of this chapter briefly highlights some of the literature on the body and the ageing body in particular. The next two sections introduce ideas from postmodernist and feminist thought, in particular exploring further the work of Grosz. I here argue that through acknowledging the embodiment of male sexed knowledge as the dominant paradigm within which the ageing body is interpreted, the relationship between knowledge, control of the body and lived experience can be further understood. This is explored further in the final section through the example of the increasing medicalization of the aged body, in particular in the USA.

## Context

There have been some excellent recent reviews of the general literature on the body; in particular the work of Frank (1990, 1991, 1992), Shilling (1993) and Turner (1984, 1991) stands forth. Yet as Shilling (1993) has pointed out, the formal recognition of the pivotal role of the body within the social sciences has been some time in the making. Furthermore, individual academic disciplines (sociology, anthropology, psychology) all seem to construct their own theory of the body, and we are still a long way from developing a grand theory of the body (even if that was desirable).

Until recently (Featherstone and Wernick 1995), while there had been extensive discussion on the body in general, the ageing body had been relatively neglected. Indeed, much gerontological research has contained discussion of the body to physical appearance (Featherstone and Hepworth 1990; Featherstone 1995). Featherstone and Hepworth (1991), for example, write vividly on the image of the mask, that tension which exists between the external appearance of face and body and functional capacities, and the experience of personal identity. Yet as the chapter will later argue, such an emphasis needs to be expanded to include the whole arena of the construction of old age. Changing physical appearance is more than a physical mask, it is the whole construction that we have placed on the chronological age of the body. It is construction/symbol/experience, the ongoing tension between the body as constructed and the body as experienced, the body as an inscribed exterior and the body as a lived interior. However, the work by Featherstone and Hepworth (1991) on the postmodern life course introduces some interesting questions. Drawing on Featherstone's work on the body in consumer culture, they argue that the postmodern world is seeing the deconstruction of the life course, with the emergent cultural tendency of some blurring of age-specific role transitions. This is supported in later life by the denial of necessary mental, physiological and sexual decline with chronological old age. As a result, loss of bodily control in extreme old age, as these facilities do naturally decline, increasingly carries the penalty of stigmatization and exclusion from mainstream social worlds. I shall return to this theme later in the chapter.

### New focus towards the body

The past decade has seen increasing focus on the body as pivotal to our understanding of social life and society. Turner (1991) has suggested three fundamental social changes which have led to this rise of interest. First, the democratization of culture and morality by the growth of mass consumption has led to the collapse of the moral apparatus of capitalism, based on Christian puritanical authority, with its religious condemnation of sexual pleasures. Second, the feminist critique of classical sociology has raised theoretical questions in which the analytical and political status of the body is pivotal. Third, the ageing of human populations has highlighted issues such as the economics of lengthening life expectancy, in particular the role of medical technology in extending this lifespan, and the ultimate ownership of control over the body. The content of this chapter has been influenced by the latter two, and by a fourth – the postmodern movement within the social sciences, which has led to a decoding and deconstruction of much that was taken-for-granted, and allowed that which was relegated to the periphery to become central.

## Postmodern thought

As Laws (1995) has succinctly summarized, four elements of postmodern thought are sympathetic to social gerontologists. First is the rejection of essentialism, the position that seeks out universal causes of social phenomenon, a rejection of meta-narratives which claim to capture universal processes and which are insensitive to local knowledge and diversity. Such searches for essential causes deny the complexity of our daily lives. Chronological, bio-logical-based age deterioration has been transformed by social structures into social and cultural signs, which are manifested in complex social relations. These relations, however, are situated in particular historical and geographical contexts, and are constantly contested and recreated in struggles over identity politics, the second and third lessons from postmodern thought. As Foucault (1983) reminded us, such identities are constructed in discourses and thereby constituted in discursive realms, rather than arising from pre-discursive subjective existence. The fourth lesson Laws suggests is that universality covers difference as well as commonality: not only should we be wary of classic dualism, which compels the search for difference, but the very idea of essential or socially constructed differences must be scrutinized. All knowledge is situated in people, places and times.

## Feminist approaches to the body

It is from within this broad framework that much recent feminist work on the body has emerged (Bordo 1989; Dallery 1989; Wiltshire 1989; Young 1990; Gatens 1991; Sawaki 1991), much of it influenced by the work of the postmodern French feminists (Kristeva 1980, 1982; Cixous 1981; Irigaray 1985). Generally these are divided between the *constructionists* and *essentialists*, but a few have attempted to bridge the gap. Most influential in this has been the work of Elizabeth Grosz, who has consistently argued that there is no necessary division between the two, but that

The body is constrained by its biological limits . . . [yet] while there must
be some kind of biological limit or constraint, these constraints are per-
petually able to be superseded, overcome through the human body's
capacity to open itself up to prosthetic synthesis, to transform or rewrite
its environment, to continually augment its powers and capacities.

(Grosz 1994: 187–8)

## The body as hinge

As an alternative perspective which incorporates both approaches, Grosz
(1993: 196) has argued that 'the body can be regarded as a kind of hinge or
threshold between a psychic or lived interiority and a more sociopolitical exte-
riority that produces interiority through the inscription of the body's outer
surface.' This interpretation has emerged from what she identifies as the two
broad approaches to theorizing the body critically. The first is *inscriptive*,
whereby the body is conceived 'as a surface upon which social law, morality,
and values are inscribed . . . a social, public body' (Grosz 1993: 196), a concept
heavily influenced by Nietzsche, Foucault and Deleuze; the second is the
phenomenological *lived body*, the body's internal or psychic inscription
derived from Freudian and Lacanian psychoanalysis.

Whereas psychoanalysis and phenomenology focus on the body as it is
experienced and rendered meaningful, the inscriptive model is more
concerned with the processes by which the body is marked, scarred,
transformed and written upon or constructed by the various regimes of
institutional, discursive, and non-discursive power as a particular kind
of body.

(Grosz, 1993: 196–7)

The body thus becomes a text, a system of signs to be deciphered, a system of
messages which constructs movement into behaviour, creating meaning and
function within the social system. 'Bodies *speak*, without necessarily talking,
because they become coded with and as signs. They speak social codes. They
become *intextuated*, narrativised; simultaneously, social codes, laws, norms and
ideals become *incarnated*' (Grosz 1993: 199; original emphasis). Yet continually
within this inscribed body is the lived body, the located body, the internalized
image, the primary experience of space and presence. Grosz argues that these
two approaches (inscriptive/lived) act to provide the concepts required to problematize some of the major binary categories defining the body: inside/outside,
subject/object, active/passive. She further argues that these pairs can be

problematized by regarding the body as the threshold or borderline
concept that hovers perilously and undecidably at the pivotal point of
binary pairs. The body is neither – while being both – the private or the
public, self or other, natural or cultural, psychical or social, instinctive
or learned, genetically or environmentally determined.

(Grosz, 1994: 23)

Yet in dissolving oppositional categories we cannot simply ignore them. 'This
is neither historically possible nor even desirable in so far as these categories
must be engaged with in order to be superseded' (Grosz 1994: 24).

## The concept of the 'other'

While there is clearly debate within feminist literature over the position and relevance of the concept of binary oppositions, within the confines of contemporary Western thought, self-conception in terms of dichotomous relationships has prevailed. In terms of these binary categories which govern Western rational thought, these pairs function in lateral arrangements, with one pair dominant over the other. Thus male/female is aligned with mind/body. Yet just as the body is the subordinated or excluded term in relation to mind, female in relation to male, so a series of binary others have similar negatives associated with them: straight/queer, white/black, young/old. A dominant theme in modern feminist discourse concerning the body is the embodiment of the 'other'. Queers[1] are defined by sexuality and thus have bodies, straights do not; blacks are defined by the colour of the skin and thus have bodies, whites do not. Feminists have long argued that those at the periphery (that is, not white, young, heterosexual etc.) are defined in terms of the 'other' – not white, not male, not heterosexual, not young. Yet such categories relate directly to the self as body: it is our bodies that are not white, our bodies that are not male, our bodies that are not heterosexual, our bodies that are not young, and it is the tension between the constructed lives of these 'not' bodies, which are imposed from without, and the experiential lives of these lived bodies that creates the person. This is an important concept, and one we shall return to later in the chapter.

## Defining a feminist critique of the ageing body

Enlarging on this theme, Grosz has argued that knowledge itself is sexed and, within contemporary thought, is male. However, she argues that the masculinity or maleness of knowledge remains unrecognized as such because there is no *other knowledge* with which it can be contrasted. We are here discussing the traditional knowledge of power, that of the sciences, humanities, social sciences, that of law and medicine, that associated with ideological and political thought.[2] This is not to exclude other knowledge, in particular the oral, intimate, private knowledge. Yet one can say that in general male knowledge until recently dominated the written culture of Western civilization, while female knowledge tended to be oral.

> Men take on the roles of neutral knowers, thinkers and producers of thoughts, concepts or ideas only because they have evacuated their own specific forms of corporeality and repressed all traces of their *sexual* specificity from the knowledges they reproduce . . . Many features of contemporary knowledges . . . can be linked to man's *disembodiment*, his detachment from this manliness in producing knowledge or truth.
>
> (Grosz 1993: 204–5)

Furthermore, men have been able to rationalize their domination of the production of knowledge by claiming that their interests are universal and sexually neutral. This has been possible through the constructed correlation of men with the category *mind* and women with *body*, the latter taking on the function of representing the *natural*. 'By positioning women as the *body*, [men] can project themselves and their products as *disembodied*, pure, and unconta-minated' (Grosz 1993: 209). This is not the result of a male conspiracy to create knowledges in their own image, but rather the result of the social meanings, values and knowledges marked upon the male body from infancy. Drawing on the work of Irigaray (1985), Grosz (1993: 208) argues that our under-standing of this system of knowledge is not limited to representations of women, but rather 'must include the elision of any *maleness* or masculinity in the perspectives and enunciative positions constitutive of knowledge.'

The work of both Irigaray and Grosz thus demands that we at least recog-nize the sexualization of all knowledges, acknowledge the sexually particular positions from which knowledges emanate and by which they are interpreted and used. Again, this is not necessarily to imply biological determinism or essentialism. That men and women experience their bodies differently has long been recognized (Sawaki 1991) (though not always acknowledged); what is key is that the *interpretation* of these experiences is *socially constructed*. Indeed, while there has been an extensive debate over sex and gender between the essentialists and social constructionists, Shilling (1993) has recently pointed out that bodies are simultaneously constructed and real: the distinc-tion between and acknowledgement of sex and gender is required by both camps. Grosz (1993, 1994) herself argues that sexual differences, like class and race differences, are bodily differences, but these are not immutable or bio-logically preordained, but are experienced through the medium of the body.

## Control and sexually situated knowledge

This insight is clearly not confined to gender discourse; there are clear state-ments of relevance for other problematic and contested relationships, includ-ing that of age. Two broad themes for those interested in ageing and later life are here explored. First, gerontologists and those interested in age and ageing need, as do all those working in the social sciences and humanities (and indeed 'natural' sciences and beyond), to acknowledge the implications of sexed knowledge. Such an acknowledgement that contemporary knowledge is sexed and male is not constraining but rather liberating, in that it allows the possibility of other knowledges. The implications of this are far reaching and far beyond the scope of this discussion, yet such recognition is the first step in the liberation of contemporary reason.

The second theme I wish to discuss in more depth, as it is specific to later life. This is the notion of embodied and disembodied knowledge, of male and female sexed knowledge, and the implications of this for our understanding of the position of the ageing body. We shall explore this further in relation to concepts of control, in particular control over the body. Control under the dominant system of knowledge can be directly related to the gendered experi-ence of the body. This operates from within and without. We all have a degree of control over our own bodies by the virtue of inhabiting them; yet through various discourses of power others also control our bodies for and on behalf of us.[3] As Douglas (1966) long ago pointed out, sexually differentiated bio-logical processes and the bodily emissions concerned with these processes are signified in all cultures. Yet the element of control that men and women have over these emissions is different and significant. For the experience of control is learnt in the first place from the body, and the experience of living within a body. Thus male seminal emissions are under the control of the male. He can generally determine when he wishes these to occur. The varied and complex emissions of women – menstruation, lactation and even childbirth itself – are not under her direct control. She cannot determine and control the timing of the flow. Menstrual blood flows at will on a predetermined corporeal schedule; breast milk descends in reaction to the other, the baby; natural childbirth occurs at the control of the body, technological childbirth at the control of others. We should perhaps here note that technology attempts to control these female emissions – women are given the pill to control and regulate menstrual flow, breast milk substitutes negate the flow from the breast, elective caesarean or induction allows control over the timing of the reproductive process.

However, as all bodies age, control as defined through male experience is reduced: incontinence, weeping orifices, bed sores, lack of control over limbs. Thus, as male bodies age, so this essential control over bodily emission starts to fail. Urinary incontinence is widespread among very old men owing to the enlargement of the prostrate, impotence spreads (Evans 1991). Male representations of female bodies as leaking and draining has been defined as a key cultural concept behind patriarchal control (Kristeva 1982). These same bodily representations are used to construct the models of later life, perpetuating what Elias (1978) refers to as the degradation of loss of bodily control with extreme old age.

Yet this is all based on one system of control as defined in order to allow the male relationship with his body to be one *of* control. Control, like power, is just a matter of situated perception and definition, and care can be read as a discipline. As both Frank (1991) and Kleinman (1988) have noted in relation to illness, infirm people desire not only care for their bodily needs, but also to be recognized in their condition, and for this condition to be acknowledged as fully human; and as Cole (1993) has so vividly pointed out, so do older people in the last years of their lives. Similarly, as with illness, the ageing body finds itself progressively unable to express itself in conventional codes. Sometimes, with the right kind of support, new codes can be developed, but these too may have only a limited duration (Dreher 1987; Giles and Coupland 1991). It can thus be argued that if absolute control of the body, defined through male experience, was not the overarching notion of adulthood, then the natural lack of control associated with extreme later life would not be so stigmatized.[4]

## A feminist understanding of the medicalization of the ageing body

The medicalization of the ageing body has attracted much attention in recent years, and various suggestions have been offered, ranging from the economic imperative (Estes 1979; Estes and Binney 1988; Estes and Swan 1993) to the fulfilment of scientific and technological endeavour (Cassel and Neugarten 1991). I should like to develop a new understanding based on the concept of sexed knowledge and control. Drawing on the work of Foucault (often critically), Sawaki (1991) has highlighted the relationship between knowledge and power, and the increasing medicalization of disciplinary normalization. Thus definitions of mental and physical health, medical and clinical surveillance, and technological and surgical interventions become crucial to other disciplining forces. Sawaki (1991) suggests that disciplinary technologies, such as advanced medical technologies, control the body through techniques that simultaneously render it more useful and more docile. They operate 'by producing new objects, generating and focusing individual and group energies, and establishing bodily norms and techniques for observing, monitoring, and controlling bodily movements, processes and capacities.'

This feminist perspective, developed in relation to the new reproductive technologies and control of women's bodies, is of particular relevance to our understanding of the medicalization and control of the *ageing* body. For as these medical disciplines isolate specific types of deviancy and disease in the body, so they construct new norms of healthy and successful ageing. As Kitwood's (1990, 1993; Kitwood and Bredin 1992) work on the construction of dementia has so vividly pointed out, in constructing the living death of Alzheimer's disease, the norm of extreme late life is relocated once again to the realms of younger healthy norms; in denying that progressive senility may be but one aspect of the normal ageing body, the young body is again projected into old age as the norm. Following Foucault's (1979) concept of disciplinary technologies, we see that control is attained by producing new norms of later life based on a medical solution to physical and mental decay. There may be different ways of defining the problem, offering new solutions, but all threaten to become submerged under the rubric of medical authority. Thus medical technologies define, reproduce and discipline both the construction and experience of old age. Reread within a feminist framework, this is part of a continuous attempt to retain control within a body that is defined in terms of the concept of the neutral/male body.

While this is not to deny liberal compassion behind such endeavours, it is also clear that in some Western countries in particular, the notion of advancing life through medical control has perhaps reached beyond the moral imperative (Estes 1979; Cassel et al. 1992). While it is possible to produce a myriad of data from the USA exploring the increasing medicalization of old age there (see Evans 1991 for an excellent review of the medical data), nothing is more vivid in its portrayal of the reality of this obsessive control of the last years of later life than Avorn's (1986) allegorical account (a 'clinical vignette') of the life of 'Oliver Shay', based on his experiences as a US physician.

'Oliver Shay was born into a lower-middle-class household at the turn of the century.' After a healthy adult life, Mr Shay came down with bacterial pneumonia at 67. Managed successfully in an intensive-care unit, he was discharged in good health less than two weeks after admission.

Two years passed, and Mr Shay began to notice pressing left-sided chest pain when he exerted himself, a condition that worsened steadily over time. Cardiac Catheterization revealed that he had a near-total narrowing of one of the main coronary arteries, which, if allowed to progress, would likely result in death within a few years. Mr Shay was scheduled for an elective coronary artery bypass operation, which he underwent successfully at age seventy-three. Six years after the operation, Mr Shay began to notice increasing pain in his left hip when he walked or climbed stairs. X-rays revealed advanced degenerative arthritis, and he underwent an elective total replacement of his hip joint. Within eight months of the operation, he was dancing at his granddaughter's wedding, and proclaimed, 'I feel like a new man!'

On the day of his seventy-ninth birthday, Mr Shay suddenly suffered a cerebrovascular accident (stroke), leaving him severely paralysed on his right side, unable to swallow, feed himself or walk.

Two days later, a nurse found him lying in bed immobile, unresponsive, and pallid. He had no pulse and was not breathing. A cardiac-arrest emergency was announced over the hospital paging system, and within minutes, closed-chest cardiac massage was implemented by the resuscitation team, a tube was placed in his windpipe to facilitate breathing, and he was attached to a respirator. Electric defibrillation and a variety of intravenous medications followed, and within thirty minutes Mr Shay once again had a normal heartbeat and blood pressure. The respirator was detached after he was moved to the intensive-care unit, and within five days he was transferred out of intensive care. Within two more weeks, impeccable nursing care and aggressive rehabilitation efforts restored Mr Shay to a point at which he could be discharged from the hospital to a skilled-care nursing home.

After living in the nursing home for two years with essentially no improvement in his paralysis and speech disorder, Mr Shay was noted to have episodes of falling, at least two of which resulted in broken bones and admission to the orthopaedic service of his local hospital . . . A cardiologist suggested that degeneration of the heart's conduction system was responsible for Mr Shay's repeated falls, and a permanent cardiac pacemaker was implanted.

Three years later, at 84, Alzheimer's disease was diagnosed. Four years later, at 88, blood tests revealed a major electrolyte imbalance, and a diagnosis was made of chronic renal failure. The family requested that he be put on haemodialysis (an artificial kidney machine) for the remainder of his life. This was done, and although he remained paralysed, and suffering from the increasing dehabilitation of Alzheimer's disease, his physical condition remained relatively stable for the next three years, until he developed severe abdominal pain at age 91.

He was sent to the emergency room of the nearest hospital where a rupturing aortic aneurysm was diagnosed, and he was rushed into surgery. After five hours in the operating room, he was transferred in very critical condition to the surgical intensive unit where he remained for ten days with a variety of complications, and then died.

Clearly, the tremendous medical advances of the twentieth century allowed considerable extension of Oliver Shay's healthy life. Yet one can argue that such an inscription of ordered control upon the suffering body also raises false hopes and denies the ultimate death. As Cole (1993: 239) has stated, 'we need to criticize liberal capitalist culture's relentless hostility to physical decline and its tendency to regard health as a form of secular salvation.' Yet the dominant biomedical ideal of successful ageing in the USA remains maximum physiological functioning (Cassel 1986; Rowe and Kahn 1987; Cassel and Neugarten 1991), though there is some limited evidence that this may be changing in some quarters (Brody 1995). While more physicians are accepting the patient's right to dignity in death, and the hospice movement is spreading, progress in the USA is still extremely slow, and currently fewer than 4 per cent of the US population die in hospices (Christakis 1996).

> By transforming health from a means of living well into an end in itself, 'successful' ageing reveals its bankruptcy as an ideal that cannot accommodate the realities of decline and death. To create genuinely satisfying ideals of ageing, we will have to transcend our exclusive emphasis on individual health and find renewed sources of social and cosmic connection.
>
> (Cole 1993: 239)

One interpretation of this extreme use of medical services is that it aims to keep the ageing body disembodied – that is, young/male. We find evidence of this in Cole's (1993) analysis of the emergence of the 'scientific management of ageing' in nineteenth-century America.

> Though seemingly gender-neutral, the search for normal ageing had a decidedly masculine flavor. Working in their new research laboratories, male scientists searched for the cause of ageing and the means of preventing senility. These men were often ageing themselves, and personal concern about declining influence, sexual potency, and productivity is sometimes evident in their writings. They sought a 'normal' old age that contained an unstated ideal of health or maximum functioning – the 'good' old age of Victorian morality.
>
> (Cole 1993: 199–200)

In our frame, they sought to retain disembodied control. As we have earlier discussed, at the philosophical level feminists have argued that women are always embodied, men are not. Yet I argue that this only pertains while men remain *not* the 'other' – for example, not black, not gay, not disabled and not old. *Men become embodied as they age.* Under patriarchal knowledge systems, while women throughout their lives cannot escape the construction of their bodies, men are enabled by this system of knowledge to deny the body for much of their lives. It is only in later life that men, like women, through the experience of the experiential and constructed body, are forced to recognize the 'other' as a defining force in their own construction and experience. Reread in the frame of sexed knowledge, embodiment and control, what Cole's ageing scientists were seeking was to retain disembodied control for themselves and for their fellow *men*.

## Conclusion

This chapter has argued that much can be learnt by those interested in later life from some of the new ideas emerging from feminist theory on the body. In particular, the concept of *sexed knowledge* and its relationship to notions of *control* over and management of the body can be enlightening. It has suggested that while physiological changes associated with later life clearly occur within a range of chronological ages, ultimate physical decline and death are the inevitable consequence of extreme old age. It is only when such mental and physical changes are fully recognized as a normal and respectable component of the human condition that the current tension between spirit and body will be resolved. Feminist theories of control and the body may help in forming a new concept of later life which fully accepts loss of bodily control, rejects the stigmatization of the declining body, and acknowledges the possibility of peace between meaning and control, symbol and experience, thus allowing the frailty of extreme later life to be fully integrated into mainstream social experience.

## Notes

1 Queers here refers to non-straight heterosexuals and thus includes gays (homosexuals), bisexuals, transvestites and heterosexuals engaged in alternative practices (see Berlant and Freeman 1993).
2 Grosz (1993) restrains her discussion to the knowledges of the social sciences and humanities; Irigaray (1985) has extended this further to include other traditional knowledge.
3 Such disciplinary regimes for 'normalizing' the body have been extensively explored in the work of Foucault, though he has been criticized by feminists for ignoring in the main the sexed nature of the bodies controlled under the power regimes and the sexed nature of the bodies constructing the knowledge enabling such disciplining.
4 This is not to argue that women find bodily ageing any less problematic than men do, for they have also grown older within the framework of a male knowledge system.

## References

Avorn, J. (1986) Medicine: the life and death of Oliver Shay, in A. Pifer and L. Bronte (eds) *Our Aging Society*. New York: Norton, 283–98.
Berlant, L. and Freeman, E. (1993) Queer nationality, in M. Warner (ed.) *Fear of a Queer Planet*. Minneapolis: University of Minnesota Press, 193–229.
Bordo, S. (1989) The body and the reproduction of femininity: a feminist appropriation of Foucault, in A. Jaggar and S. Bordo (eds) *Gender/Body/Knowledge*. New Brunswick, NJ: Rutgers University Press, 13–33.
Brody, J. (1995) Postponement as prevention in aging, in R. Butler and J. Brody (eds) *Delaying the Onset of Late-life Dysfunction*. New York: Springer.
Cassel, C. (1986) The meaning of health care in old age, in T. Cole and S. Gadow (eds) *What Does It Mean to Grow Old?* Durham, NC: Duke University Press, 179–98.
Cassel, C. and Neugarten, B. (1991) The goals of medicine in an aging society, in R. Binstock and S. Post (eds) *Too Old for Health Care*. Baltimore: Johns Hopkins University Press, 75–91.

Cassel, C., Rudberg, M. and Olshansky, J. (1992) The price of success, *Health Affairs*, Summer, 87–99.

Christakis, N. (1996) The US hospice movement: unpublished paper presented to the Demographic Workshop, University of Chicago.

Cixous, H. (1981) The laugh of the Medusa, in E. Marks and I. de Courtivron (eds) *New French Feminisms*. Amherst: University of Massachusetts Press, 245–64.

Cole, T. (1993) *The Journey of Life*. Cambridge: Cambridge University Press.

Dallery, A. (1989) The politics of writing the body: ecriture feminine, in A. Jaggar and S. Bordo (eds) *Gender/Body/Knowledge*. New Brunswick, NJ: Rutgers University Press, 52–67.

Dreher, B. (1987) *Communication Skills for Working with Elders*. New York: Springer.

Douglas, M. (1966) *Purity and Danger*. London: Routledge and Kegan Paul.

Elias, N. (1978) *The Civilizing Process*. Oxford: Blackwell.

Evans, R. (1991) Advanced medical technology and elderly people, in R. Binstock and S. Post (eds) *Too Old for Health Care*. Baltimore: Johns Hopkins University Press.

Estes, C. (1979) *The Ageing Enterprise: a Critical Examination of the Social Policies and Services for the Elderly*. San Francisco: Jossey-Bass.

Estes, C. and Binney, A. (1988) Towards a transformation of health and ageing policy, *International Journal of Health Services*, 18, 69–82.

Estes, C. and Swan, J. (1993) *The Long Term Care Crisis*. Newbury Park, CA: Sage.

Evans, R. (1991) Advanced medical technology and elderly people, in R. Binstock and S. Post (ed.) *Too Old for Health Care*. Baltimore: Johns Hopkins University Press.

Featherstone, M. (1982) The body in consumer culture, *Theory, Culture and Society*, 1, 18–33.

Featherstone, M. (1995) Post-bodies, aging, and virtual reality, in M. Featherstone and A. Wernick (eds) *Images of Aging: Cultural Representations of Later Life*. London: Routledge.

Featherstone, M. and Hepworth M. (1990) Images of ageing, in J. Bond and P. Coleman (ed.) *Ageing in Society*. London: Sage.

Featherstone, M. and Hepworth, M. (1991) The mask of ageing and the post-modern lifecourse, in M. Featherstone, M. Hepworth and B. Turner (eds) *The Body: Social Process and Cultural Theory*. London: Sage, 371–89.

Featherstone, M. and Wernick, A. (eds) (1995) *Images of Aging: Cultural Representations of Later Life*. London: Routledge.

Foucault, M. (1979) *Discipline and Punish*. New York: Vintage Books.

Foucault, M. (1983) The subject and the power, in H. Drefuss and P. Rabinow (eds) *Michel Foucault: Beyond Structuralism and Hermeneutics*. Chicago: University of Chicago Press.

Frank, A. (1990) Bringing bodies back in: a decade review, *Theory, Culture and Society*, 7(1), 131–62.

Frank, A. (1991) For a sociology of the body: an analytical review, in M. Featherstone, M. Hepworth and B. Turner (eds) *The Body: Social Process and Cultural Theory*. London: Sage, 36–102.

Frank, A. (1992) *At the Will of the Body: Reflections on Illness*. Boston: Houghton Miller.

Gatens, M. (1991) Corporeal representation in/and the body politic, in R. Diprose and R. Ferrell (eds) *Cartographies: Poststructuralism and the Mapping of Bodies and Spaces*. Sydney: Allen and Unwin, 79–87.

Giles, H. and Coupland, N. (1991) *Language: Contexts and Consequences*. Buckingham: Open University Press.

Grosz, E. (1993) Bodies and knowledges: feminism and the crisis of reason, in L. Alcoff and E. Potter (eds) *Feminist Epistemologies*. New York and London: Routledge.

Grosz, E. (1994) *Volatile Bodies*. Bloomington and Indianapolis: Indiana University Press.

Irigaray, L. (1985) *The Sex which Is Not One*. Ithaca, NY: Cornell University Press.

Kitwood, T. (1990) The dialectics of dementia: with particular reference to Alzheimer's disease, *Ageing and Society*, 10, 177–96.

Kitwood, T. (1993) Towards a theory of dementia care: the interpersonal process, *Ageing and Society*, 13, 51–67.

Kitwood, T. and Bredin, K. (1992) Towards a theory of dementia care: personhood and well-being, *Ageing and Society*, 12, 269–87.

Kleinman, A. (1988) *The Illness Narratives*. New York: Basic Books.

Kristeva, J. (1980) *Desire in Language*. New York: Columbia University Press.

Kristeva, J. (1982) *Powers of Horror: an Essay on Abjection*. New York: Columbia University Press.

Laws, G. (1995) Understanding ageism: lessons from feminism and postmodernism, *The Gerontologist*, 35(1), 112–18.

Martin, E. (1989) *The Woman in the Body*. Boston: Beacon Press.

Rowe, J. and Kahn, R. (1987) Human ageing: usual and successful, *Science*, 237, 143–9.

Sawaki, J. (1991) *Disciplining Foucault*. New York and London: Routledge.

Shilling, C. (1993) *The Body and Social Theory*. London: Sage.

Turner, B. (1984) *The Body and Society*. Oxford: Basil Blackwell.

Turner, B. (1991) Recent developments in the theory of the body, in M. Featherstone, M. Hepworth and B. Turner (eds) *The Body: Social Process and Cultural Theory*. London: Sage, 1–35.

Wilshire, D. (1989) The uses of myth, image and the female body in re-visioning knowledge, in A. Jaggar and S. Bordo (eds) *Gender/Body/Knowledge*. New Brunswick, NJ: Rutgers University Press, 92–114.

Young, I. (1990) *Throwing Like a Girl and Other Essays in Feminist Philosophy and Social Theory*. Bloomington: Indiana University Press.

**PART III**

---

# Concluding analysis

---

ANNE JAMIESON AND CHRISTINA VICTOR

# Theory and concepts in social gerontology

As explained in our introduction, the issues discussed in this book relate to two broad areas of discourse. One concerns *epistemological aspects*, highlighting different positions regarding the status of knowledge. The other relates more directly to concepts of *ageing and later life*. In this chapter we shall deal with each in turn.

## Epistemological issues in gerontology

### Gerontology and disciplines

This book has brought together contributions concerned with theoretical and conceptual development. Taken as a whole, the book is multidisciplinary, and many of the chapters are interdisciplinary, defying any clear disciplinary categorization. It must be emphasized, of course, that the focus in this volume is upon *social* aspects of ageing, and thus does not include contributions from biomedical sciences.

Literature, history, sociology, social policy, geography and anthropology are all represented in this volume, but it is difficult and perhaps irrelevant to assign each chapter solely to one of these. Disciplinary boundaries among the social sciences in general have become increasingly blurred, and conventional definitions of the disciplines are only of limited use. Definitions by object of study would, for example, see history as being about the past, geography about space, sociology about social relations, literature about fiction and so on. Definitions by method would, for example, distinguish between history as an idiographic science, focusing on 'the unique', sociology as nomothetic, searching for patterns and generalizations.

As Troyansky's chapter illustrates, historical data are used sociologically to throw light on general questions related to the meaning of life course stages, of retirement and its implications, and the social factors affecting the role of older people in different societies. Similarly, Zeilig's chapter on literature discusses its use as a source for the social gerontologist in search of generalizable understanding of later life. The two chapters on paintings and photographic images are also predominantly sociological in so far as they consider representations in the arts as 'social data' which can be given meaning within a wider sociological framework. Indeed, the interest in 'images', whether from popular culture or from the arts, has long been central in gerontology because of its concern to deconstruct and challenge existing perceptions of age and older people.

The boundaries between gerontologists, whether in terms of what they study or in terms of the methodologies used, are therefore not clear-cut – or rather, they are not primarily disciplinary boundaries. This is not to say that there are no differences and at times conflicting views and perspectives, but to a large extent these cut across disciplines and reflect differences regarding the purpose of gerontology and the nature of knowledge and science. We will consider what this involves, first by taking a closer look at what in much American literature is referred to as critical gerontology, and second by commenting on postmodernism as an epistemological position.

## Critical gerontology

An understanding of 'the spirit' of critical gerontology is perhaps best achieved by examining one of its sources of inspiration, to which Achenbaum refers in his chapter, i.e. the Frankfurt School of critical theory. The Frankfurt Institute, set up in 1930 and associated with Max Horkheimer, Theodor Adorno and Herbert Marcuse, raised some profound questions about the role of the social sciences in society, questions which were particularly pertinent given the rise of fascism in Europe during the 1930s, but which remain important. The ideas of the early Frankfurt writers were taken up and developed in the late 1960s by Habermas. His exposition of what he sees as the relation between *knowledge* and *interest* has been of crucial influence, and provides a useful basis for an understanding of the meaning of critical gerontology (Habermas 1970).

Summarized very briefly, Habermas distinguishes between three types of inquiry or knowledge seeking, each driven by a distinct interest or goal. The first interest is inherent in the natural sciences and is essentially technical; that is, to look for regularities enabling prediction and thereby *control*. The second interest is inherent in the historical interpretative – hermeneutic – sciences and is the quest for *understanding or meaning*. Third, the social sciences, or sciences of action, are guided by an interest in *emancipation*. This, according to Habermas, means that social science does not stop at the search for regularities, but goes one – very important – step further: it tries to discover how far such regularities are ideologically based and therefore changeable. Thus 'ideology critique' is an essential part of social science, as is its close relation between theory and *practice*: that is, human beings are *reflexive* beings; understanding can bring about change (emancipation).

From the point of view of critical theory, positivism in the social sciences is criticized for imitating the natural sciences and confining itself to a search for regularities of human behaviour and technical solutions – a concern with means rather than goals. Thus it ignores the link between theory and practice, and hence excludes itself from a search for meaning and from a critique of ideology. It ignores the development of free communication and does not search for alternatives to existing patterns of behaviour.

Critical theory is essentially 'negative critique', as it is called, i.e. a critique of the limitations of positivist science and of the values of instrumental rationality inherent in mainstream theorizing; rather than positive critique, i.e. a statement of an alternative theory. It is perhaps best described as a set of notions which have to varying degrees inspired scholars in the humanities and social sciences.

The concept of *critical gerontology* should be seen in this context. Achenbaum's account of critical gerontology, its background and influences, suggests very clearly that it would be misleading to talk of a specific 'school' of critical gerontology. A wide variety of writings are seen to come under the umbrella of 'critical gerontology', as illustrated further in the volume edited by Cole *et al.* (1993). It is, however, possible to discern a number of distinct strands in the US critical gerontology.

First, there are critiques of an *epistemological* nature, i.e. of positivism and its 'physics envy', to use the words of Achenbaum in this volume. What is criticized is the view that the 'truth' about ageing can be measured 'objectively', and the drive to control the process of ageing through the acquisition of such 'knowledge'. Yet, in parallel with Habermas's arguments, critical gerontology does not exclude an empirical search for patterns of social relations, as Achenbaum acknowledges very clearly (Bookstein and Achenbaum 1993). Other proponents of critical gerontology also stress the need for measurement: 'we need measurement – of morale, retirement rates, caregiver burden and all the other issues discussed by social gerontology. But we ought not to remain uncritical about what measurements or responses mean' (Moody 1993: xxiv).

In short, as Habermas also argues, measurement is necessary but not sufficient. It needs to be complemented with two other endeavours: the search for an *understanding* of the meaning of the patterns of activities, and a critique of their ideological basis. Thus, the two other distinct features of critical gerontology are the *humanistic* (hermeneutic) approach and the *political* approach. The former puts 'life' into statistics, and attempts to understand the meaning of ageing through literature, personal accounts etc. The latter emphasizes a critical examination of the production of ageing and gerontological knowledge, including the effects of class, gender and race, with the aim of empowering older people. The task of empowerment of older people is emphasized even more strongly by other writers. Thus Minkler (1996), in her discussion of the contributions of critical gerontology, places a great deal of emphasis on social responsibility and advocacy as being part of the task of critical gerontology. All three concerns – epistemological critiques, humanistic perspectives and political critiques – are not confined to gerontology, but, as illustrated by Achenbaum, are perhaps more developed in other areas, like feminist research.

Critical gerontology can perhaps best be described as an awareness of and a commitment to the emancipatory interest inherent in the social sciences as stated by Habermas – an aspiration rather than a body of knowledge or theory. No wonder therefore that Phillipson (1996), in his review of Cole *et al.* (1993), notes that 'the lack of clarification of the idea of critical gerontology is a problem' (p. 265).

It is debatable whether the sharp lines which appear to have been drawn between 'mainstream' and 'critical' gerontology in the USA are paralleled elsewhere. Certainly, the term 'critical gerontology' does not appear often in gerontological writings in Britain, where many aspects of what Achenbaum highlights as critical gerontology are part of mainstream gerontology.

Thus interdisciplinarity is a feature of much social gerontology, and seems to be increasing, as evidenced not only in this volume, but in much writing published in Britain and elsewhere in Europe. Secondly, the humanistic tradition of qualitative work, including biographical approaches, is well established in Britain (Thompson 1988; Bornat 1993). The interest in literature has been limited, but is growing, as illustrated by Zeilig's contribution to this volume. Jefferys's personal account, included in our collection, is another example of what Achenbaum advocates when he says that 'too few of our successful elders . . . have offered introspective commentaries on their lives' careers' (p. 24). Third, feminist perspectives have for some time had considerable influence in critical analyses of the lives of older women, their material circumstances, social networks and involvements in care (e.g. Finch and Groves 1988; Arber and Ginn 1995). Fourth, as others have pointed out (Walker 1987), macro-theory or political gerontology has played a prominent part in the development of British gerontology.

One of the dimensions which Achenbaum sees as part of critical gerontology is the culture of ageing, which, if studied critically, can yield insights relevant to effective policy implementation. In this respect critical gerontology in Britain is perhaps 'lagging behind' American thinking. Blakemore's chapter in this volume highlights the lack of attention paid to the comparative dimension, and he is particularly critical of the use of culture and ethnicity which is confined to minority experiences. He advocates a view of both culture and ethnicity which invites us to examine the constructed and contested nature of identity in the so-called 'majority' community. This involves the study of ageing in Britain which does not take for granted the cultural context of the older English, Scottish or Welsh person, and which could examine more explicitly than before how that context differs from the cultures or cultural contexts. Furthermore, 'ethnicity' can only be defined by an examination of ethnic *relations*, for ethnic identity arises from a process of social interaction, mutual labelling and sometimes political conflict. Blakemore therefore suggests that, in addition to the more critical examination of the role of culture, we should also turn our gaze to the ways in which an ethnic dimension in relationships between older people and others may either exaggerate or reduce inequalities of power and status: for instance, in the case of an older white English person being treated by an Asian doctor, or when – at a group or community level – an 'ethnic community' is created as a pressure group in the welfare system or in local politics, as with the emergence of an 'Afro-Caribbean' community in Britain.

## Postmodernism

Several of the contributions to this volume adopt an epistemological position which can best be described as postmodernism. (This is not to be confused with 'postmodernity', a concept used by many to describe contemporary society and aspects of contemporary society, like the 'postmodern' life course. This does not imply a particular epistemological position.) Like critical gerontology, postmodernism as an epistemology encompasses a diversity of positions. Although some, like Achenbaum, see affinities between the two, there is an important difference, highlighted, for example, by Cole (1993), when he refers to Habermas as one of the most forceful opponents of extreme postmodernism. Critical gerontology, in so far as it is at all associated with critical theory, is based on notions of enlightenment and reason, as distinct from ideology and suppressed dialogue. Within postmodernist theory, on the other hand, the distinction between reason and ideology, or between 'essence' and 'appearance', is problematic, because:

> The world comes to us in the shape of stories. Anything we try to substitute for a story is, on closer examination, likely to be another story . . . Every narrative simultaneously presents and represents a world, that is, simultaneously creates or makes up a reality and asserts that it stands independent of that same reality . . . narrative seems at once to reveal or illuminate a world and to hide or distort it.
>
> (Sarup 1988: 141–2)

The implication of this position is that analysing the world means analysing discourse (or texts or narratives), as social (and other) phenomena exist in discourse. Discourse analysis represents an alternative both to the positivist notion that there is an objective truth 'out there' to be discovered, and to the ethnomethodologists' position that everything is subjective. In other words, there is not seen to be a distinction between the subjective and the objective world. This, for example, is what Harper refers to when she stresses the view that identities are constructed in discourses and do not exist outside of these. Furthermore, she suggests that 'texts' need not be just words, and that the living *body* itself can be seen as a text, which is part of the lived experience and not separate from it. Similarly, Laws, in her chapter on the *built environment*, conceives of it as a kind of text, which because it is experienced contributes to the construction of social life. Fairhurst treats *memories* in the same way. Thus she argues that they are not just to be seen as a means to an end, or as something different from 'real experience'. Hence she rejects a 'correspondence theory of truth' – that is, an approach which would 'test' the 'truth' of memories against some 'objective' events – and favours a 'coherence theory of truth', which examines discourse in relation to other texts. Finally, Latimer, in her account of *professional discourse* in a hospital setting, stresses that such discourse is not to be criticized as based on myths or unreal representations of older people. Rather, they should be analysed as 'lived experiences', in which older people are produced and reproduced as a lived category. Her aim therefore is to explain the existence of such categories.

Postmodern thinking is far from being a neatly defined school of thought, and it is beyond the scope of this volume to consider the different positions and contradictions associated with it. However, the rejection of the distinction between 'concepts' and 'reality' is important, as it makes references to 'data' as distinct from 'theory' meaningless. This does not necessarily have to entail a totally relativist position, whereby all stories are seen as being of equal value. A coherence criterion (that is, looking for consistency between texts) is just as rigorous as a correspondence view of 'truth' (that is, looking for concepts which correspond to the 'objective' world). For example, Jefferys (Chapter 11), in 'telling her story', is right to question whether this has more than anecdotal or illustrative value. Individual stories, in parallel with fictional accounts, cannot in themselves be taken as representations of generalizable social phenomena. They have to be interpreted or *contextualized*, and when they are understood in the context of other texts or analyses, including perhaps the reader's own experience, the possible strengths of such accounts become manifest. Thus Jefferys's account is both a personal account and a sociological commentary. It is also a powerful demonstration that social theory is a lived experience. Not only does it remind us that we, the gerontologists, are ourselves ageing, but it also suggests that gerontological insight is part of and therefore informs our understanding of our own life course.

In devoting attention to some of the very complex epistemological issues, our aim has been one of clarification. In addition, however – even though epistemological positions vary, and aspects of critical theory conflict with aspects of postmodern theorizing – it is possible to draw out from this what in our view ought to be the common concern in social gerontology; that is, a concern to be *critical*. We need to be critical first of everyday discourses – public or private – of age and older people. Second, and equally important, is the need to be critical of gerontological discourse, its concepts and measurements. To be critical means pointing out inconsistencies between discourses, whether expressed in words or figures, and uncovering implicit assumptions underlying arguments about ageing and older people. It also means constantly reviewing existing discourses and seeking new ways of conceptualizing ageing issues.

## Conceptualizing ageing and later life

*Ageing and later life: what are we studying?*

As social gerontologists wishing to develop theory we are constantly faced with the problem of defining – and perhaps therefore of justifying – what we are actually studying. We are forever on our guard against applying age categories, against referring to 'the elderly'; we are at pains to point to the diversity of the experience of ageing, to the importance of class, gender and culture. So what is the distinctiveness of our subject? Does it make sense at all to attempt to theorize age? Certainly, as stressed in the chapter by Bytheway, we must be critical of our own as well as others' concepts of age, older people and life course stages. A great deal of gerontology, therefore, has become engaged in deconstructing and critically analysing existing discourses or 'images' of ageing and older people.

The notion of the life course perspective has for some time been part of the gerontology discourse, witnessed, for example, in an earlier book published under the auspices of the BSG (Arber and Evandrou 1993). This perspective is not a theoretical framework, and its merits and weaknesses are debatable (Walker 1987; Blaikie 1992). It is best viewed as a map of orientation, suggesting important points to look out for on the road to an understanding of ageing. Three points appear of particular significance. First, it is an attempt to get beyond an age-based definition of the subject matter of gerontology, emphasizing movement through the life course, and the meaning of different life stages, rather than relying on slippery concepts like 'old age' or 'the last stages of life'. Second, the perspective postulates some association between earlier and later stages of the life course, and as such provides a basis for biographical studies. For this reason it has been criticized for neglecting the search for macro-theory (Walker 1987); but this need not be so. Thus a third aspect of the perspective is its stress on placing individual ageing experience in the context of changing social structures (Hareven and Adams 1982).

A focus on 'the life course' or 'adult life' rather than 'older people' or 'later life' may help us to overcome the problem of age-based definitions, but some would argue that it diverts attention from the oldest members of our societies and the last stage of life. But is this not a risk worth taking? Should we as gerontologists not be more concerned to understand the meaning and social implications of age, if not at all stages of the life, at least from the age of maturity? If we do not think so, we should perhaps consider more carefully why not.

### Retirement, consumerism and the politics of ageing

Much of the literature in social gerontology developed around the notion of *retirement* and its role in the social construction of old age. The meaning of retirement has changed significantly, and its usefulness as a basis for a critique of ageism has become increasingly problematic, as debated in the chapter by Higgs. Ever since it was first put forward, the *structured dependency* theory has been criticized for viewing retired people and therefore older people as a homogeneous category, all suffering social exclusion due to retirement (Phillipson 1982; Johnson 1989; Thomson 1992). The growing visibility of healthy, active and affluent retired people has led to a shift in focus away from production and non-productivity towards patterns of *consumption* as a crucial factor in the construction of later life. Laws's chapter is one such example. Using the American Sun City retirement communities as her case material, she argues that Sun City 'is a landscape to be consumed'. It is the spatial representation of a particular retirement culture, a particular construction of retired life as happy, communal activity, protected from, yet in touch with, the surrounding community. She is further arguing that the identities manifest through these retirement communities have been created by business interests, recognizing a market niche and thus promoting a particular lifestyle.

As in the case of structured dependency theory, the focus appears to be on capitalism, but it has shifted from employment considerations or personnel departments to marketing and sales. This raises the old question of how far patterns of consumption are shaped by economic interests, and how far they reflect people's real wishes. Consumerism, as argued by Hepworth (1996), could be seen as representing increasing freedom from traditional constraints, as a way of enabling the expression of diversity and choice. Thus a focus on consumption may help to dispel some of the traditional ageist assumptions surrounding older members of our societies. Sojourn in a Sun City village may not be entirely to everyone's taste (nor of course within everyone's means), but to some it may well represent a preferred lifestyle, and an extension of previous forms of living. A focus on the consumption of different forms of living space would certainly seem to provide further understanding of the diversity of old age, and the cultural differences rooted in earlier life course experiences – experiences which are highly variable within particular societies as well as between countries and over time.

However, the notion of consumerism as a key to an understanding of the plight of older people has its limitations. Certainly, recent trends in the welfare discourse in Britain suggest that the language of consumerism itself and its penetration of policy debates highlight divisions within the older generation. The chapter by Higgs argues that, increasingly, British social policy under the Tory regime has moved from a rights-based to a consumer-based notion of citizenship. The clients of the welfare state are becoming 'customers', exercising 'choice', with procedural rather than substantive rights. Self-reliance is given more importance than state protection. Under such circumstances, Higgs argues, the likelihood of a specific politics of old age is limited, since the 'third agers' will increasingly distance themselves from the 'fourth agers', thus denying 'old age'.

The consumer culture of late modern (or, as some would say, 'postmodern') society reflects a shift in the conception of motivation as arising from *necessity* towards one emphasizing *desire* (Hepworth 1996). Herein lies one of its dangers, that of ignoring all those whose 'consumption' is guided more by necessity than desire. Concepts such as inequality, social exclusion and deprivation are still important. The question remains whether there are any significant features associating such notions with *age*. Structured dependency theory, as already pointed out, suffers the weakness of homogenizing older people. Furthermore, exclusion from the labour market is not confined to older people only. Uncertainty and insecurity has become a feature of the late modern economy, affecting people at all stages of their life course. If permanent insecurity is becoming a feature of the *'modern' career*, this will have implications for the analysis of the association between social exclusion and age. In other words, a life course perspective on social policy would seem more relevant than ever. We need to understand the situation of tomorrow's as well as today's older generations.

It is also important to acknowledge the possibility that in matters of social exclusion and deprivation, age may often be of less importance than factors such as *gender, ethnicity, education and occupation*. Jefferys's account in this volume highlights the importance of class background, and it points to some interesting issues around the notions of retirement, which deserve more attention. As someone who has been able to continue professional involvement, her confession to feeling some forms of social exclusion, therefore, needs explaining. Could it be that in our eagerness to see retirement as a source of social exclusion, we have not paid sufficient attention to the possible insight which could be derived from considering the minority who are still working at the age of 80?

Paradoxically perhaps, the distance experienced by Jefferys in relation to her younger colleagues is not entirely one which depicts her own position as less privileged. On the contrary, in stressing that her generation of academics 'do not envy our successors', who operate in a climate of contraction, unpredictability and insecurity, she highlights the importance of considering cohort-specific aspects of life course experiences, and her particular statement suggests an added meaning to the notion of the 'welfare generation'. Debates around pensions and their funding do to an extent revolve around the question of inter-generational solidarity, and whether there is a 'welfare generation' (Thomson 1992; Falkingham and Hills 1995; Johnson 1995). But we must acknowledge that differences within generations may provide much better clues to an understanding of the tensions and the sources of indifference, if not antagonism, felt by parts of the younger generation towards their elders.

The welfare discourse on the distribution of values between generations and the role of the state in generating them needs to include a *comparative dimension*. We have to acknowledge an absence of this dimension in this volume. The chapter by Higgs on citizenship and old age leads one to raise the question of how far it makes sense to theorize the politics of old age, not just because of the diversity among older people, but because of the differences which exist between societies. Just as cultural differences are important, so too are the differences between political regimes and the role played by the state, even within the modern world. The shifts in the role of the British welfare state suggested by Higgs are not taking place to the same extent or in the same ways everywhere. A consumerist, residual welfare approach is well known in the USA, whereas, at the other extreme, some of the Scandinavian welfare states still retain a Marshall type notion of social citizenship, which includes its older citizens in the social protection system. A comparative perspective is essential, therefore, and here concepts from the general social policy literature can be used as a way of understanding the politics of ageing (e.g. Esping-Andersen 1990; Sainsbury 1994; Alber 1995; Jamieson 1996).

Comparison at all levels helps us to develop a critical perspective; it helps to eliminate ethnocentricity in generalizations about the position of older people; it keeps our eyes open to what might be possible rather than accepting current policy trends as inevitable. This seems particularly important when it comes to the question of our attitudes and practices in relation to those in need of care.

## Frailty, care and the end of life

A vast amount of gerontology literature has focused on frailty in old age and questions of care provision. In social gerontology, a great deal of work is concentrated around policy and service evaluation, and some conceptual work is associated with it; for example, around the notions of dependency, need, health and disability. Among the debates about service provision the question of the respective roles of the health service and social services still figures prominently on the agenda, not only in Britain, but in most countries of the developed world. At the core of much of this debate has been a critique of the medicalization of later life, and calls for giving social care a more prominent role.

Two chapters in this volume relate to such care issues, one focusing on social care (Johnson and Bytheway), the other on health care (Latimer). Their focus is on the construction of identities in care discourse. The analysis by Johnson and Bytheway suggests that attitudes of professional carers, as presented in photographs in a much read magazine for carers, are still depicting older people in institutions as passive recipients of care, despite moves to change such attitudes. The question of what is desirable and indeed achievable in institutions is a burgeoning theme in gerontology. Institutions are increasingly places almost exclusively for people with severe impairments, partly as a result of home care policies, and partly because the pressure on health care systems is to cater only for 'medical cases', and, as Latimer says, to 'dispose of' older people.

Latimer argues that through the discourse which goes on among the professions in this setting, older patients are, in a sense, defined out of the system. Their illnesses are constructed as natural and associated with age, and rapid disposal is the prime object of their assessment. Latimer is at pains not to condemn the professionals, but instead points to the structures which lead to such behaviour, i.e. the pressures towards cost containment and increased throughput. Thus the definition of what is 'medical' is increasingly being narrowed down, enabling the hospital to push the older people out of the medical system.

While the medicalization of old age has been much criticized over the years (e.g. Binney *et al.* 1990; Jamieson 1992), the trend towards demedicalization is equally problematic. It provides justification for denying health care and even long-term care for those who actually need them. It is to a large extent the outcome of a lack of adequate alternatives, which in many countries left the health care system as the only option for older people, whether they were 'ill' or just frail. The growing pressure on health care systems has led to the situation described by Latimer. Questions around the role of health care systems are likely to continue to be of crucial importance in gerontology, not only in regard to long-term care responsibilities, but also concerning the relevance of age as a criterion for access to acute medicine. Callahan and others have added fuel to the debate among gerontologists by raising issues concerning end-of-life decisions and the role which professionals, individual old people and representatives of the state should play (Callahan 1987).

Attacks on 'life extension' endeavours and denial of death philosophies have come from different perspectives. The growing criticism has gone hand in hand with growing disillusionment with features of modern society and the belief that technical progress can solve all our problems. Some; like Harper in this volume, argue from a feminist perspective that the negative image associated with bodily frailty is owing to the dominance of male knowledge systems. Whatever the perspective, it continues to be important for social gerontology to address issues relating to bodily decline and frailty, not just as things to avoid, or to legitimize 'care needs', but as part and parcel of the ageing process. Much of gerontology has been driven by a concern to uncover the many ageist assumptions underlying so many debates and policies. In doing so there has perhaps been a tendency to overdo the arguments that 'age does not matter'. The signs in gerontology now are that age is beginning to be taken seriously as something which relates as much to distance from death as to distance from birth. Frailty and death are no longer considered solely in terms of 'problems', 'burdens' and 'care needs', but as common experiences of life (Houtepen 1995; Moody 1995).

## Conclusion

Issues of ageing are studied by researchers from a variety of backgrounds. Many (though perhaps not enough) contributions to an understanding of ageing continue to be made by scholars who do not necessarily devote their entire professional life to such issues. Gerontology as a specific area of study was stimulated partly by the ageing of contemporary societies. It was partly also a response to the often peripheral status of the age dimension in mainstream scholarly activity. The dilemma for gerontology is that, while it highlights the importance of ageing as a topic, its multidisciplinarity also has to be stressed. Not only do we need to draw upon the insight and expertise of a variety of disciplines, but ageing issues can often only be understood in the contexts within which they occur. This means that contributions to the understanding of ageing cannot be expected solely from within what is labelled gerontology. At the same time, gerontologists need to ensure that ageing issues become more central in all relevant disciplines. Some would argue that the ultimate goal of its scholars is to make gerontology superfluous, either on the grounds that ageing issues cannot be understood in isolation, or on the grounds that its core mission is precisely to point to the problematic nature of the phenomenon of 'old age', and all that the term has been used to imply. In the words of Hazan (1994: 93),

> Whereas the endless pursuit of knowledge about ageing endows the phenomenon with the illusion of intelligibility, that very quest renders it unique and inexplicable. Hence the production of knowledge about ageing is self-subversive.

Whether or not we think that gerontology can or indeed should become superfluous, we are in any case a long way from this goal. There is a lot of work to be done in the task of understanding ageing and debunking myths about age. This means that essentially the task of gerontology is to be *critical*. We need to continue to count, measure and evaluate, but we also need to keep the subject alive through theoretical and conceptual developments, aiming always to find new ways of thinking about it. We hope that this book will make a contribution to these enterprises.

# 186   Concluding analysis

## References

Alber, J. (1995) A framework for the comparative study of social services, *Journal of European Social Policy*, 5(2), 131–49.

Arber, S. and Evandrou, M. (eds) (1993) *Ageing, Independence and the Life Course*. London: Jessica Kingsley Publishers.

Arber, S. and Ginn, J. (eds) (1995) *Connecting Gender and Ageing*. Buckingham: Open University Press.

Binney, E.A., Estes, C.L. and Ingman, S.R. (1990) Medicalization, public policy and the elderly: social services in jeopardy?, *Social Science and Medicine*, 30(7), 761–71.

Blaikie, A. (1992) Whither the third age?, *Generations Review*, 2(1), 2–4.

Bookstein, F.L. and Achenbaum, W.A. (1993) Aging as explanation: how scientific measurement can advance critical gerontology, in T. Cole, W.A. Achenbaum, P.L. Jakobi and R. Kastenbaum (eds) *Voices and Visions of Aging: toward a Critical Gerontology*. New York: Springer.

Bornat, J. (1993) *Reminiscence Reviewed: Perspectives, Evaluations, Achievements*. Buckingham: Open University Press.

Callahan, D. (1987) *Setting Limits: Medical Goals in an Aging Society*. New York: Simon and Schuster.

Cole, T. (1993) Preface, in T. Cole, W.A. Achenbaum, P.L. Jakobi and R. Kastenbaum (eds) *Voices and Visions of Aging. Toward A Critical Gerontology*. New York: Springer.

Cole, T., Achenbaum, W.A., Jakobi, P.L. and Kastenbaum, R. (eds) (1993) *Voices and Visions of Aging. Toward a Critical Gerontology*. New York: Springer Publishing Company.

Esping-Andersen, G. (1990) *The Three Worlds of Welfare Capitalism*. Cambridge: Polity Press.

Falkingham, J. and Hills, J. (1995) *The Dynamics of Welfare. The Welfare State and the Life Cycle*. London: Prentice Hall/Harvester Wheatsheaf.

Finch, J. and Groves, D. (eds) (1988) *A Labour of Love: Women, Work and Caring*. London: Routledge and Kegan Paul.

Habermas, J. (1970) Knowledge and interest, in D. Emmet and A. MacIntyre (eds) *Sociological Theory and Philosophical Analysis*. London: Macmillan.

Hareven, T. and Adams, C. (eds) (1982) *Ageing and Life Course Transitions*. London: Tavistock.

Hazan, H. (1994) *Old Age: Constructions and Deconstructions*. Cambridge: Cambridge University Press.

Hepworth, M. (1996) Consumer culture and social gerontology, *Education and Ageing*, 11(1), 19–30.

Houtepen, R. (1995) The meaning of old age and the distribution of health-care resources, *Ageing and Society*, 15(2), 219–42.

Jamieson, A. (1992) Home care in old age: a lost cause?, *Journal of Health Politics, Policy and the Law*, 17(4), 879–98.

Jamieson, A. (1996) Ageing in place: opportunities and constraints in the development of home care services, in P. Hennessy (ed.) *Caring for Frail Elderly People: Policies for the Future*. Paris: OECD.

Johnson, M. (1995) Interdependency and the generational compact, *Ageing and Society*, 15(2), 243–65.

Johnson, P. (1989) The structured dependency of the elderly, in M. Jefferys (ed.) *Growing Old in the Twentieth Century*. London: Routledge.

Johnson, P. and Falkingham, J. (1992) *Ageing and Economic Welfare*. London: Sage.

Minkler, M. (1996) Critical perspectives on ageing: new challenges for gerontology, *Ageing and Society*, 16(4), 467–87.

Moody, H.R. (1993) Overview: what is critical gerontology and why is it important?, in T. Cole, W.A. Achenbaum, P.L. Jakobi and R. Kastenbaum (eds) *Voices and Visions of Aging: toward a Critical Gerontology*. New York: Springer.

Moody, H.R. (1995) Ageing, meaning and the allocation of resources, *Ageing and Society*, 15(2), 163–84.

Phillipson, C. (1982) *Capitalism and the Construction of Old Age*. London: Macmillan.

Phillipson, C. (1996) Interpretations of ageing: perspectives from humanistic gerontology, *Ageing and Society*, 16(3), 359–69.

Sainsbury, D. (ed.) (1994) *Gendering Welfare States*. London: Sage.

Sarup, M. (1988) *An Introductory Guide to Post-structuralism and Postmodernism*. Hemel Hempstead: Harvester Wheatsheaf.

Thompson, P. (1988) *The Voice of the Past*. Oxford: Oxford University Press.

Thomson, D. (1992) Generations, justice and the future of collective action, in P. Laslett and S. Fishkin (eds) *Justice between Groups and Generations*. New Haven, CT: Yale University Press.

Walker, A. (1987) Ageing and the social sciences: the North American way, *Ageing and Society*, 7(2), 235–41.

# Index

## AGEISM

### Bill Bytheway

Ageism has appeared in the media increasingly over the last twenty years.

- What is it?
- How are we affected?
- How does it relate to services for older people?

This book builds bridges between the wider age-conscious culture within which people live their lives and the world of the caring professions. In the first part, the literature on age prejudice and ageism is reviewed and set in a historical context. A wide range of settings in which ageism is clearly apparent are considered and then, in the third part, the author identifies a series of issues that are basic in determining a theory of ageism. The book is written in a style intended to engage the reader's active involvement: how does ageism relate to the beliefs the reader might have about older generations, the ageing process and personal fears of the future? To what extent is chronological age used in social control? The book discusses these issues not just in relation to discrimination against 'the elderly' but right across the life course.

The book:

- is referenced to readily available material such as newspapers and biographies
- includes case studies to ensure that it relates to familiar, everyday aspects of age
- includes illustrations – examples of ageism in advertising, etc.

*Contents*
*Part 1: The origins of ageism – Introduction: too old at 58 – Ugly and useless: the history of age prejudice – Another form of bigotry: ageism gets on to the agenda – Part 2: Aspects of ageism – The government of old age: ageism and power – The imbecility of old age: the impact of language – Get your knickers off, granny: interpersonal relations – Is it essential?: ageism and organizations – Part 3: Rethinking ageism – Theories of age – No more 'elderly', no more old age – References – Index.*

158pp    0 335 19175 4 (Paperback)    0 335 19176 2 (Hardback)

## ELDER ABUSE IN PERSPECTIVE

### Simon Biggs, Chris Phillipson and Paul Kingston

What is elder abuse? How can it be explained and understood? Why now? What can be done about it?

Elder abuse is now recognized as a serious social problem on both sides of the Atlantic and Australia. Our understanding and responses to it will have profound implications for the quality of older people's lives and their place in society.

*Elder Abuse in Perspective* examines how the mistreatment of older people is defined, theorized and researched. It places the problem in its social and historical context, giving special attention to forms of abuse within families, communities, and institutions like hospitals and residential homes. The book looks at issues around training and elder abuse, and explores the most effective methods of intervention and prevention.

*Elder Abuse in Perspective* challenges many commonly held assumptions and provides new insight into elder abuse and neglect. It is perhaps the first book in recent years to provide a critical and reflective analysis of this growing social issue. It is an essential addition to the library of practitioners, researchers and students of old age.

### Contents
*Introduction – Historical perspectives – Theoretical issues – Definitions and risk factors – Social policy – Family and community – Institutional care and elder mistreatment – Training and elder abuse – Interventions – Conclusion: the challenge of elder abuse – References – Index.*

160pp     0 335 19146 0 (Paperback)     0 335 19147 9 (Hardback)

## CONNECTING GENDER AND AGEING
A SOCIOLOGICAL APPROACH

### Sara Arber and Jay Ginn (eds)

- How do the social effects of ageing over the life course interact with gender, giving rise to changed gender roles and relationships?
- How do women's and men's sense of their identity change with increasing age?

*Connecting Gender and Ageing* challenges the assumption that gender can be treated as static over the life course, highlighting the differential social effects of ageing on women's and men's roles, relationships and identity. The early chapters address the question of linking gender and age within sociological theory, outlining alternatives and introducing new ideas to integrate these two dimensions of social stratification.

Contributors use a feminist perspective to explore the impact of ageing on gender roles in the workplace and in retirement; in marital and other relationships; in community support networks and in older women's own perceptions. A range of research approaches are used, including qualitative studies giving a voice to older women. A concluding chapter draws out the implications of the book. A clear writing style and the inclusion of chapters from North America and Europe makes this book accessible to an international readership.

### Contents

*'Only connect': gender relations and ageing – Ageing, gender and sociological theory – Theorizing age and gender relations – Conformity and resistance as women age – Gendered work, gendered retirement – Choice and constraint in the retirement of older married women – The married lives of older people – 'I'm the eyes and she's the arms': changes in gender roles in advanced old age – Mutual care but differential esteem: caring between older couples – Gender roles, employment and informal care – Gender and elder abuse – Gender and social support networks in later life – Connecting gender and ageing: a new beginning? – References – Index.*

### Contributors

Sara Arber, Janet Askham, Mirian Bernard, Errollyn Bruce, Mike Bury, Lori D. Campbell, Jay Ginn, Doris Ingrisch, Catherine Itzin, Anne Martin Matthews, Julie McMullin, Chris Phillipson, Hilary Rose, Anne Scott, Julie Skucha, G. Clare Wenger, Terri Whittaker, Gail Watson.

224pp     0 335 19471 0 (Paperback)     0 335 19470 2 (Hardback)